Aesthetic and Functional Alterations of the Labia Majora

Pablo Gonzalez Isaza
Editor

Aesthetic and Functional Alterations of the Labia Majora

A Comprehensive Guide to Clinical Approaches and Procedures

Springer

Editor
Pablo Gonzalez Isaza
Obstetrics and Gynecology Urogynecology Minimally invasive Surgery
Hospital Universitario San Jorge
Pereira, Colombia

Soranus Center for Funtional and Regenerative Urogynecology
Pereira, Colombia

ISBN 978-3-031-97404-5 ISBN 978-3-031-97405-2 (eBook)
https://doi.org/10.1007/978-3-031-97405-2

This Springer imprint is published by the registered company Springer Nature Switzerland AG
The registered company address is: Gewerbestrasse 11, 6330 Cham, Switzerland

Foreword

In a world where aesthetics and functionality are increasingly complexly intertwined, women's health and well-being have taken center stage in contemporary medical discourse. Attention to labia majora alterations, from both an aesthetic and functional perspective, has gained prominence in the field of gynecology, challenging professionals to address these concerns with a comprehensive and up-to-date approach.

Dr. Pablo Gonzalez Isaza, a pioneer in cosmetic genital surgery in Colombia and a leader in the training of new specialists around the world, presents this book with a fundamental work that not only reflects on the anatomy and alterations of the labia majora but also offers a practical framework for the treatment of these conditions. With an accumulated experience of 15 years and the support of an extensive academic and clinical background, Dr. Pablo Gonzalez Isaza dives into the complexities of female anatomy, proposing a structured classification that promises to revolutionize the way we approach aesthetic and functional concerns in this delicate area.

This book becomes an indispensable tool for gynecologists, aesthetic surgeons, and all those involved in female health care, providing clear guidelines and an algorithmic approach that will allow professionals to take a comprehensive approach to the care of the female anatomy.

Luksenburg Center, Montevideo Uruguay
S.M.I. (Servicio Médico Integral),
Montevideo, Uruguay

Ariel Luksenburg

Contents

Contributors

Red Alinsod Institute of Restorative and Cosmetic Gynecology, Davis, CA, USA
Alinsod Institute PLLC, Dallas, TX, USA

Pablo Gonzalez Isaza Obstetrics and Gynecology, Urogynecology Minimally Invasive Surgery, Hospital Universitario San Jorge, Pereira, Colombia
Soranus Center for Funtional and Regenerative Urogynecology, Pereira, Colombia

Ana Maria Gutierrez Private Operating Room Calculaser, Pereira, Colombia

Gustavo Leibaschoff Obstetrician and Gynecologist Private Practice, Dallas, TX, USA

Gustavo Parra Profamilia Clinic, Manizales, Colombia

Michael A. Reed Institute of Restorative and Cosmetic Gynecology, Davis, CA, USA
Alinsod Institute PLLC, Dallas, TX, USA

Diana Lorena Vélez Rizo Gynecologist and Obstetrician Universidad de la Sabana, Cundinamarca, Colombia
Colposcopy and Cervical Pathology Universidad Nacional de, Bogotá, Colombia
Laser and Gynecologic Functional Aesthetic Surgery AGEOC Association of Colombian Aesthetic Gynecologists, Bogotá, Colombia
Laser Applications in Gynecology Universidad Nacional de, Bogotá, Colombia
Master in Clinical Sexology, University of Valencia, Valencia, Spain
Urological and Reconstructive Gynecology of the Pelvic Floor National University of Colombia, Bogotá, Colombia
Gynecologist in Dr. Diana Velez Rizo Advanced Gynecology, Fundación Cardioinfantil and Clínica de la Mujer, Bogotá, Colombia

Enrique Tang-Villanueva Radiologist, MSK and Soft Tissue Interventionist, Pereira, Colombia

Chapter 1
Introduction

Pablo Gonzalez Isaza

Female genital cosmetic surgery is still considered a controversial area, and there is a lack of clear medical indications, nomenclature, and guidelines.

Most scientific data available is related to the treatment of labia minora hypertrophy; limited information is published regarding the treatment of labia majora skin laxity, deflation, and fat loss which impacts the vulvar appearance [1]. Today there is increasing demand for treatment of the labia majora related to the normal process of aging such as decrease of volume, tone, and vascularization of labia majora (Fig. 1.1) [2]. Patients frequently report a bulging sensation and discomfort during sport activities and entry dyspareunia. Fasola et al. proposed a standardized classification in three stages for labia majora related to the degree of hypotrophy, appearance of the skin, and subcutaneous structures and associated functional complaints from patients [3]. The aesthetic desires by women regarding the labia majora were categorized in 2022 in the International Journal of Urogynecology where Stage 0 desires no alteration, Stage I desires augmentation, and Stage II desires reduction with added suffixes for laxity (L) and asymmetry (A). This system is very useful because it addresses aesthetic and functional concerns from patients [4].

The most common procedures described for labia majora are augmentation with autologous fat or fillers [2, 5], augmentation with dermal grafts and labia minora transposition [6, 7], and labia majora reduction by a variety of surgical techniques [8, 9] or by tightening the skin with energy-based devices [10]. Sometimes certain clinical conditions require a combined approach [11].

The main purpose of this book is to offer cosmetic gynecology practitioners around the world, structured protocols for the treatment of functional and aesthetic

P. Gonzalez Isaza (✉)
Obstetrics and Gynecology, Urogynecology Minimally Invasive Surgery,
Hospital Universitario San Jorge, Pereira, Colombia

Soranus Center for Funtional and Regenerative Urogynecology, Pereira, Colombia

P. Gonzalez Isaza (ed.), *Aesthetic and Functional Alterations of the Labia Majora*, https://doi.org/10.1007/978-3-031-97405-2_1

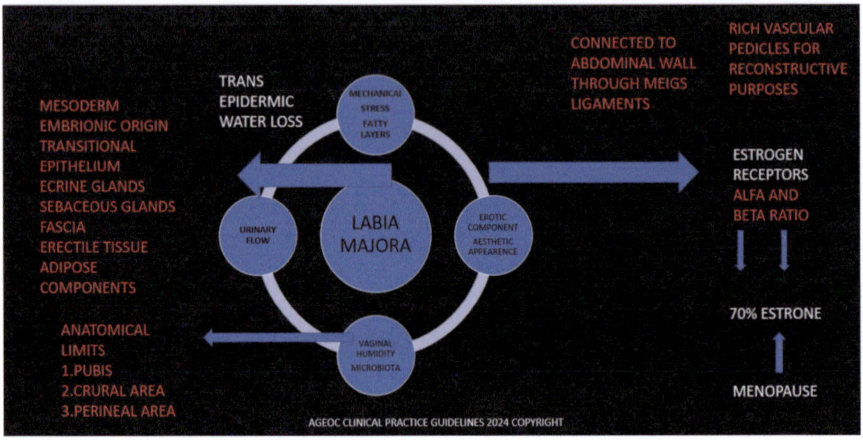

Fig. 1.1 Labia majora function and changes

problems of the labia majora based on anatomy, clinical conditions, therapeutic options, and competences.

References

1. Lowe J, Black KI. Female genital cosmetic surgery. Aust N Z J Obstet Gynaecol. 2021;61(3):325–7. https://doi.org/10.1111/ajo.13363. PMID: 34109617
2. Zerbinati N, Haddad RG, Bader A, Rauso R, D'Este E, Cipolla G, Calligaro A, Gonzalez P, Salvatore S, Serafin D. A new hyaluronic acid polymer in the augmentation and restoration of labia majora. J Biol Regul Homeost Agents. 2017;31(2 Suppl. 2):153–61. PMID: 28702976.
3. Fasola E, Gazzola R. Labia Majora augmentation with hyaluronic acid filler: technique and results. Aesthet Surg J. 2016;36(10):1155–63. https://doi.org/10.1093/asj/sjw083. Epub 2016 May 30. PMID: 27241363.
4. Developed by the Joint Writing Group of the International Urogynecological Association and the American Urogynecologic Society. Joint Report on Terminology for Cosmetic Gynecology. Int Urogynecol J. 2022;33(6):1367–1386. https://doi.org/10.1007/s00192-021-050107. Epub 2022 May 23. PMID: 35604421.
5. Jabbour S, Kechichian E, Hersant B, Levan P, El Hachem L, Noel W, Nasr M. Labia Majora augmentation: a systematic review of the literature. Aesthet Surg J. 2017;37(10):1157–64. https://doi.org/10.1093/asj/sjx056. PMID: 28449124.
6. Salgado CJ, Tang JC, Desrosiers AE 3rd. Use of dermal fat graft for augmentation of the labia majora. J Plast Reconstr Aesthet Surg. 2012;65(2):267–70. https://doi.org/10.1016/j.bjps.2011.07.010. Epub 2011 Jul 30. PMID: 21803669.
7. Karabağlı Y, Kocman EA, Velipaşaoğlu M, Kose AA, Ceylan S, Cemboluk O, Cetin C. Labia Majora augmentation with De-epithelialized labial rim (Minora) flaps as an auxiliary procedure for labia Minora reduction. Aesth Plast Surg. 2015;39(3):289–93. https://doi.org/10.1007/s00266-015-0474-z. Epub 2015 Apr 3. PMID: 25835708.
8. Hunter JG. Labia Minora, labia Majora, and clitoral Hood alteration: experience-based recommendations. Aesthet Surg J. 2016;36(1):71–9. https://doi.org/10.1093/asj/sjv092. Epub 2015 Oct 24. PMID: 26499942.

9. Mottura AA. Labia majora hypertrophy. Aesth Plast Surg. 2009;33(6):859–63. https://doi.org/10.1007/s00266-008-9260-5. PMID: 19205794.
10. González Isaza P, Rizo DV, Garibay I, Galvan R. The role of bipolar radiofrequency (Bprf) as a mechanism of bio-stimulation for the treatment of Vulvo-vaginal laxity: a novel approach. Int J Clin Exp Med Res. 2021;5(3):367–76. https://doi.org/10.26855/ijcemr.2021.07.022.
11. Miklos JR, Moore RD. Simultaneous labia minora and majora reduction: a case report. J Minim Invasive Gynecol. 2011;18(3):378–80. https://doi.org/10.1016/j.jmig.2010.12.013. PMID: 21545962.

Chapter 2
Historical Aspects of Labia Majoraplasty Surgery: A Personal Perspective

Red Alinsod

My first introduction to labial surgery was in 1985 as a third-year medical student at Wilford Hall Medical Center in San Antonio, Texas. Kenneth Hancock, MD, gynecologic oncologist, was instrumental in helping me learn gynecologic anatomy and introduced me to vulvar surgeries. I was fascinated by radical vulvectomies. I saw him teach his residents. Dr. Hancock was fresh out of his Gynecologic Oncology Fellowship at University of Texas MD Anderson Cancer and Tumor Institute (no MD Anderson Cancer Center). "Anderson" was well known for his aggressive and radical surgeries headed by Felix Rutledge, MD. He was known for Total Pelvic Exenterations (aka Exents) for advanced cervical and uterine cancer. Dr. Hancock became instrumental in writing a letter for me to obtain my residency at Loma Linda University Medical Center who had three gynecologic oncologists. Robert Wagner, MD, and Elden Keeney, MD, were graduates of MD Anderson. The chairman of the department was Alan King, MD, also a gynecologic oncologist from Memorial Sloan Kettering Medical Center in New York. My path was set. I was going to be a gynecologic oncologist.

In my third year of residency at Loma Linda I heard about competitive fellowships that were going to be started by the two biggies: The Rutledge Fellowship by MD Anderson and the Galloway Fellowship by Memorial Sloan Kettering. With great support and encouragement by my Loma Linda faculty I was accepted to both. I chose to be a Rutledge Fellow, the first one ever, and off I went to Houston. That was 1988, the year L.A. Dodger Kirk Gibson hit that walk off home run against the Oakland As. I was post call and watching it when it happened that evening. My month at MD Anderson was an eye opener. I had never seen any program work their residents harder and with full support and dedication. Their stated goal was to build the finest

R. Alinsod (✉)
Alinsod Institute PLLC, Dallas, TX, USA

Institute of Restorative and Cosmetic Gynecology, Davis, CA, USA
e-mail: red@gynflix.com

P. Gonzalez Isaza (ed.), *Aesthetic and Functional Alterations of the Labia Majora*, https://doi.org/10.1007/978-3-031-97405-2_2

surgeons with the best hands to be the boss and run departments. It is a bit intimidating for sure. I met Dr. Rutledge who was retired and on his third wife but who came to all the meetings and even showed up for the endless number of Exents done by the Fellows. I was completely overwhelmed being among legends like David Gershenson, MD, Taylor Wharton, MD, Michelle Follen, MD, and Mitchell Morris, MD.

The exenterations removed all the reproductive organs, bladder, anus, vulva, and bowel, and we created pouches for urine and stool. There was an "Above Team" that took care of the abdominal hysterectomies and bowel and bladder surgery. There was a "Below Team" that did the complete vulvectomies and made neovaginas out of gracilis muscle. I made sure I spent most of my time as part of the Below Team. I loved that they let this third-year resident do the fellows work to recreate labias and vaginas from the inner thigh tissue. I was in my element. The staff was very encouraging and pushed me to pursue pelvic surgery. There was no urogynecology fellowship at that time, so the next logical step was to see if infertility surgery was for me. So, I went to Yale to do a 1-month elective in Reproductive Endocrinology in my senior year of residency. I was completely unimpressive. The chairman at the time was the famous Alan DeCherney, MD. I worked exceptionally hard with the fellows doing inseminations and IVF. I was in meetings almost every day doing Case Planning with the team headed by Dr. DeCherney. At the end of my rotation, I went up to Dr. DeCherney and thanked him for his mentorship and he said "and who are you again?" I realized reproductive endocrinology (REI) was not for me.

As disappointed as I was for my lackluster performance at Yale's REI division, I was blessed to meet one of the most modest and brilliant man I had ever encountered E. Albert Reece, MD. He was a Maternal Fetal Medicine Doctor attending along with John Hobbins, MD. They are the giants who deciphered the causes and treatments for gestational diabetes. Dr. Reece was a devout Seventh Day Adventist Christian and taught me the ropes of academia counseling me to ALWAYS make sure to thank the Attending Staff personally and with letters, so they do not forget me. He encouraged me not to be narrow-minded and just automatically go to MD Anderson for my GYN ONC Fellowship, so he introduced me to Peter Schwartz, MD, and Setsuko Chambers, MD, who later offered me the one fellowship position that was to start in July 1990. I accepted. Then disaster struck. The First Gulf War was about to heat up, so the Air Force told me I had to be on active duty and that my deferral for starting my Gynecologic Oncology Fellowship at Yale was rescinded. I was heartbroken notifying Dr. Schwartz that I was not able to be his 1990 Fellow. This disappointment turned into excitement as I served for 4 years at George and Nellis Air Force Base.

I had the privilege to care for the women of the military and retirees. I ran the Gynecology Department and did hundreds of pelvic reconstruction cases. I was surprised to see a demand for labial reduction surgery even then in the early 1990s. So, I did them with both electrocautery and my CO_2 laser. I lasered so many venereal wart lesions then. I started using the laser on the labia minora and majora not just for venereal warts. Air Force salaried soldiers and their wives, retirees, and dependents could not afford to see a plastic surgeon in town, so I was more than happy to do their surgeries labial surgeries and prolapse and tightening surgeries. In my eyes it was an easy surgery when compared to the exenterations I had been doing with the teams at MD Anderson.

After my Air Force career, I entered private practice in Los Angeles and for a medium-sized multispecialty group. The field of urogynecology was starting to grow rapidly, and this really was what I wanted to pursue. From 1994 to 2004 I worked with industry and designed slings and mesh repair kits and surgical tools. I did a few labiaplasty surgeries because it was not a thing back then. Urogynecology was starting to be "The Thing" that gave birth to unofficial fellowship programs like Ostergaard's at UC Irvine. Laparoscopy was booming with the rise of Marco Pelosi II and III, Harry Reich, John Miklos, C.Y. Liu, and David Redwine. I saw gynecology change slowly from being a specialty for vaginal surgery to laparoscopic surgery. It made me more determined to try and retain and expand vaginal surgery and ensure it was not a lost art. I actively taught for Caldera Medical, AMS, BARD, and Ethicon. I taught the UCLA residents and eventually became the mesh repair clinical instructor for Harbor UCLA's Urogynecology Fellowship from 1997 to 2005. I focused strictly on labial and vaginal surgeries.

In 2000 I heard about David Matlock and reached out to him right after he completed his MBA at UC Irvine. He had just finished his MBA Group Project of launching the **Laser Vaginal Rejuvenation Institute of America**. His group aced it. The project became his outline for successfully launching LVRIA. He graduated his first LVRIA class soon after his MBA graduation. I heard about it and was in awe that people would pay so much money for such a course. I saw him take labiaplasty surgery and vaginoplasty surgery into the mainstream with lots of headwinds and naysayers. To this day!

I recently asked David why he even went back to school to get his MBA. He said:

> *One thing I learned about an MD, MBA, is that people look at you differently in the business world. A very good friend of mine asked "Why do you need this? You're already a good businessman," and I told him I felt that I was holding myself back. That's why I did it. In my interview with one of the professors, she was called away for a short period of time she had my essay in front of her and what I noticed was that she had highlighted, and I stated* ***I seek knowledge****. When I saw that I knew I was in. I have a whole lot of stories, my friend.*
>
> *Obviously, with any business, they're going to be critics. You had to have a thick skin and push through it. The criticism was weird, was the lack of research. There was plenty of research there because of what some of these procedures were drawing from. I knew 100% that the research would come! Therefore, I pushed forward. I was able to grow this nationally in internationally. The media came to me, and I really understood that sex sells. I've been on everything. Television shows nationally and internationally, magazines, Vogue, Harper Bazar, Cosmopolitan, Nationally, Internationally, etc., etc. So, look where we are today! I knew that's what would happen. Now it's accepted and it's International. F*** all those nay sayers in the beginning!*

David ran the first Cosmetic Gynecology courses in history in Beverly Hills starting in 2000 and said this:

> *As you may or may not know I entered it as a business venture and first secured intellectual property with a patent attorney. I trained I've 436 surgeons in over 46 countries. I would train up to 10 at a time. I did world, European, and Asian, organized by the marking*

company. Get this we were able to charge $60k per doctor. Crazy money. But I liked at it as a business deal.

Run those numbers serious money was made. Some people may have rejected for me commercializing it but that's what I learned in my MBA program. That's what the professors told us to do. Just like many grad students coming out and launching businesses.

I only trained gynecologist, plastic surgeons, and urologist. That's it. The doctor spent three days with me. One day of didactics, one day seeing me in surgery, performing the cases, and one day in the lab working on inanimate objects to simulate all the procedures. The support group putting all this together was a marketing company. A laser marketing company. It was a well-oiled machine.

I started a movement, and I was right. Let alone that I publicized it nationally in internationally with free marketing for everyone. Actually, that's why we are where we are, and I understood, and I told the media I need them, and they need me"

In the beginning, David taught Designer Laser Vaginal Rejuvenation (labiaplasty surgery) and Laser Vaginal Rejuvenation (vaginoplasty and perineoplasty). For the saggy labia majora, he initially used a wide perineoplasty technique to pull the labia majora downward to reduce the sag and draping effects but ultimately found this to be unsatisfactory. The problem of a tight introitus and potential for dyspareunia were present with this method. I asked him if his perineoplasty was his initial approach to saggy labia majora, and he said "that was one of the ways that I used to help reduce the majora. Ultimately, I didn't get the results that I wanted, and I've stopped that approach. I'm sure I showed them (his Fellows) both. The best approach is the vertical elliptical/reduction."

For the majora, I found that the best approach would be a midline vertical elliptical excision. You can do anything to reduce the length, thickness, decrease thickness with that incision. With a medial approach you can't get that and then that has the potential to fish-mouth labia minora.

Jack Pardo, MD, from Chile, one of Dr. Matlock's earliest graduates, remembers learning the midline vertical elliptical excision from Dr. Matlock. Jack's grandfather and father were tailors, and his exposure to gynecologic oncology made him secure about female genital anatomy. He did not do many vulvectomy surgeries early in his career but had the exposure to become confident in knowing where the vessels and nerves were located. To his recollection he did his own first solo "U.S. Football"-shaped labia majora excision in 2009. Here are photos from Dr. Pardo's landmark publication showing the medial incision going close to the labia minora and the pale white scar at the top of the labia majora ridge (shown with permission) (Figs. 2.1 and 2.2).

Marco Pelosi III gained valuable experience working with pelvic surgeons and gynecologic oncologists and plastic surgeons early on after residency. Again, the common thread seems to be the work with the Gynecologic Oncology specialists. Macro Pelosi III also remembers the midline vertical elliptical excisions that removed a football-shaped area of labia majora tissue on each side. However, in Dr. Pardo's recollection, the elliptical excision was horizontal going across the middle of the labia majora and when sutured "pinched" the majora to reduce the sagging.

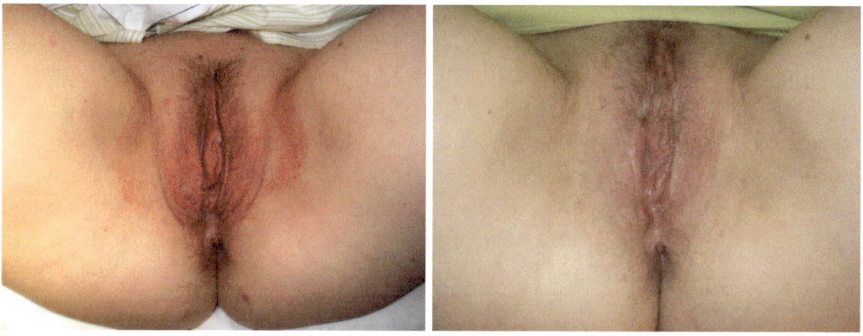

Figs. 2.1 and 2.2 Interlabial fold technique of incision before and after (shown with permission from Dr. Jack Pardo Chile)

This technique morphed into a more aesthetically pleasing vertical elliptical excision ("more banana shaped and not symmetrical" per Pardo) and changed the horizontal scar across the labia minora to a vertical scar on each majora. An American football-shaped excision of labia majora was developed by Pelosi and Pardo. The only problem was that now there was a railroad track scar on the middle of the labia majora. This was not a big problem in the days when women were not shaving everything off. However, when the days of the Brazilian waxing and laser hair removal became more prevalent, Dr. Pardo, and his colleagues, modified their techniques further and placed the medial incision closer to the labia minora to hide the scar once healed. Doctors Jack Pardo, Vicente Sola, and Paolo Ricci submitted their landmark research on 60 labia majora lifting patients on September 18, 2011, and it was published in The American Journal of Cosmetic Surgery in 2012. Patients were collected from May 2004 to June 2011. At that point in history, David held the surgical secrets close to the vest like the Chamberlains did with their obstetrics delivery forceps. I was much the same as David and did not publish any of my cosmetic gynecology techniques. Jack remembers telling David Matlock and John Miklos about an earlier publication regarding colpoperineoplasty on Acta Scandinavia that initially drew David Matlock's and John Miklos' disapproval of revealing secrets, but this turned out to be a positive attraction toward David's LVRIA program.

As comfort and experience grew with labiaplasty surgery (minora and majora and clitoral hood), Dr. Jack Pardo brought his surgeries into the office in Latin America and began teaching his surgery under local anesthesia. Dr. Michael Goodman had the same experience as he taught local anesthesia techniques worldwide for labial and vaginal cosmetic surgeries in 2010.

As David Matlock's LVRIA empire was rapidly expanding in stature and influence in the early 2000s and my pelvic surgical world focused on design of products for use in pelvic reconstructive surgery. Many of these products would ultimately be instrumental in allowing for in-office awake No IV surgeries for cosmetic gynecology. My patented Alinsod Stand Surgical Table allowed still and calm hands for delicate labial surgery. My Alinsod Scissors and pickups and clams allowed for deep pelvic reach and placement of sutures. The Lone Star Retractor allowed for vision deep into the vagina. The slings and ultralightweight mesh and dermal allografts we brought out to market helped transform urogynecology. I was in Los Angeles at this time in my career (1994–2004) and watching how successfully David and his fellows were changing the gynecology landscape. I was recruited as a urogynecologist to Laguna Beach, California, by South Coast Medical Center, who envisioned capturing the pelvic floor surgery business in the South Orange County region where the average age of women was in the mid-40 s. My vision was to combine urogynecology with cosmetic gynecology and integrate the two. So, I moved and opened shop on January 5, 2005. I did the large majority of my labiaplasty and vaginoplasty surgeries in my office and started teaching and giving courses in both urogynecologic surgery and cosmetic gynecology. My big secret was the pudendal-levator block and labial blocks with microtumescent anesthesia I had developed that allowed deep pelvic floor dissections in the office. I kept all my labiaplasty and vaginoplasty secrets and my anesthesia techniques very private and only for my Alinsod Fellows. I chose not to publish at the time but to collect and share my thousands of before and after pictures to those in search of surgical results. I had nondisclosures signed as did Dr. Matlock.

I launched my Alinsod Institute for Aesthetic Vulvovaginal Surgery training program in 2006 and started the Congress of Aesthetic Vulvovaginal Surgery (CAVS) in 2006 in conjunction with the now defunct AAOCG (American Academy of Cosmetic Gynecology). The first lecture on labia majoraplasty was at that Congress in Las Vegas with the first live course in Laguna Beach in October 2007. Prominent surgeons I had the thrill to work with in those early years were Dr. Alexander Bader in 2008, Dr. Michael Goodman in 2010, Dr. Sejal Ajmera in 2012, Dr. Christine Hamori in 2013, Dr. Amr Seifeldin in 2015, Dr. Joao Jaenisch in 2015, Dr. John Miklos, and Dr. Robert Moore in 2017. They have taught, spoken, or have published on labia majoraplasty and have been the most influential surgeons in the field of labia majoraplasty. I thank them for their contributions. One significant publication of note is the May–June 2011 article written by Miklos and Moore titled "Simultaneous Labia Minora and Majora Reduction: A Case Report," published in the *Journal of Minimally Invasive Gynecology*. Theirs is the first publication of a combination surgery involving the labia majora. I had taught this method in my fellowship program and presented it in several Congresses showing dozens of videos I call the "Universal Approach."

My first labia majoraplasty was done in the office in 2005. Looking back at all my photos and videos and reading all the available materials published show that my first photographed labia majoraplasty using the Curvilinear Labia Majoraplasty technique was on March 1, 2007. There are no sets of labia majoraplasty photos I can find that predate these photo sets. I believe these to be the very first non-cancer labia majoraplasty photos ever taken (Figs. 2.1 and 2.2). My technical modification was to hug the medial incision line to be as close to the labia minora as possible to hide the scar but not remove so much tissue that a gaping introitus appears (Figs. 2.3, 2.4, 2.5, and 2.6). Going short of this anatomical remark and leaving the scar line lateral to the minora–majora junction risking a visible white pale scar being visible.

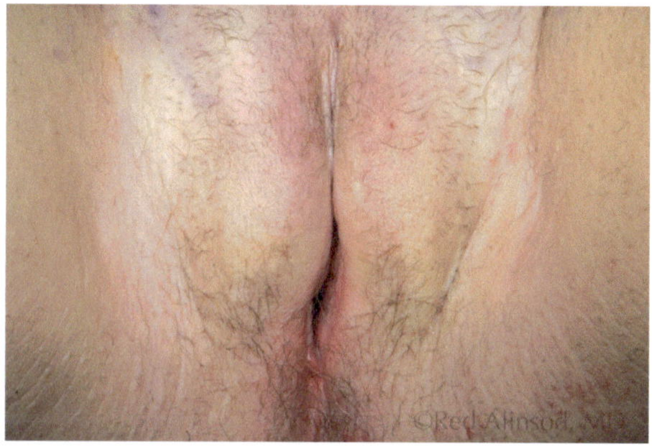

Fig. 2.3 Before labia majoraplasty

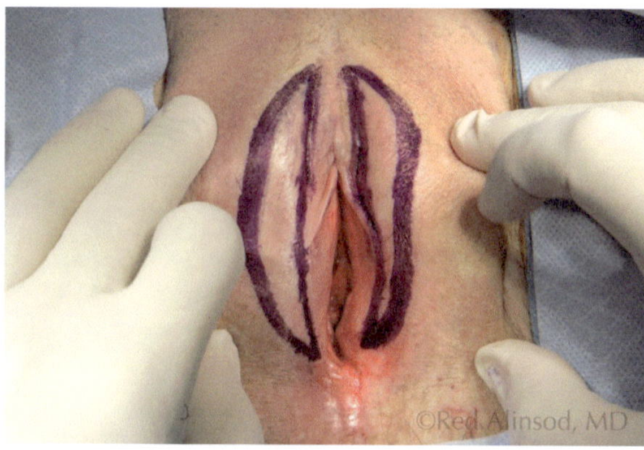

Fig. 2.4 Markings for labia majoraplasty that hug the labia minora and the clitoral hood

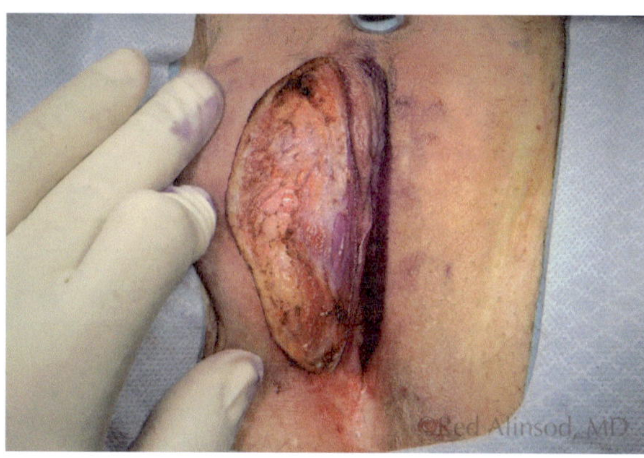

Fig. 2.5 Right Labia majora after excision

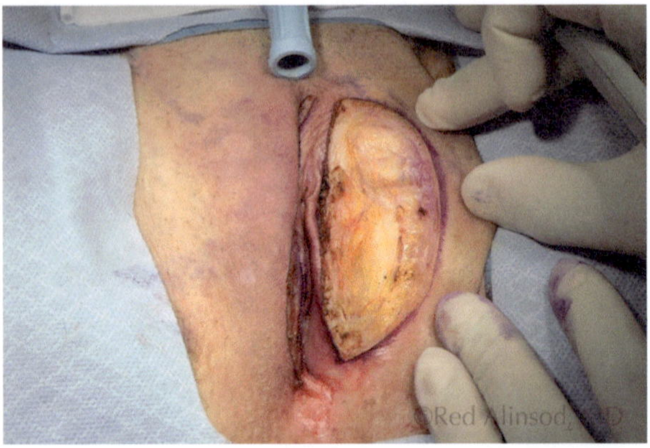

Fig. 2.6 Left labia majora after excision

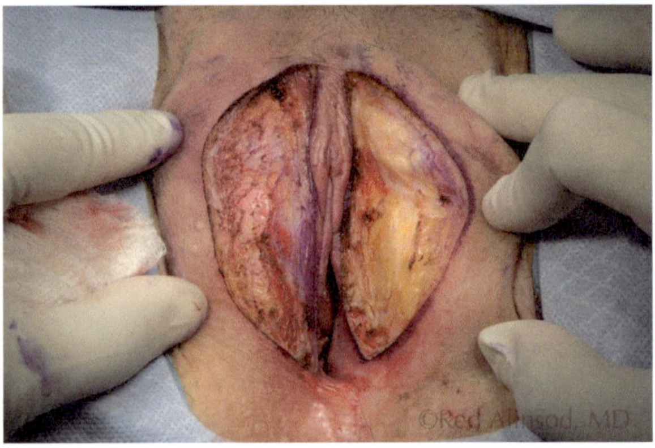

Fig. 2.7 Labia majoraplasty excision complete

Here is that case and the photos I used to teach my Alinsod Fellows (Figs. 2.7, 2.8, 2.9, 2.10, 2.11, 2.12, 2.13, and 2.14).

The second set of labia majoraplasty pictures I took were 3 weeks later on May 21, 2007, as I expanded my teaching sets as more and more surgeons were showing interest in my surgical preceptorship. Here is Case 2 that highlighted the tightening of the vagina, perineum, and labia majora.

Historically, only the skin of the labia majora is removed when doing a labia majoraplasty. When a large "Camel Toe" is present, liposuction has been tried to remove fat. It has not been very successful. In vulvar cancer surgery, the labia majora is often removed, as well as the fat with dissection done all the way to the muscles beneath the pubic ramus. Lymph node dissection is performed in these cases. This surgery has been modified to be a cosmetic labia majora reduction that includes a great deal of normal but voluminous fat (Figs.2.15, 2.16, 2.17, and 2.18). The first case of labia majoraplasty with fat pad reduction for cosmetic indications was performed in my Laguna Beach office on February 29, 2012.

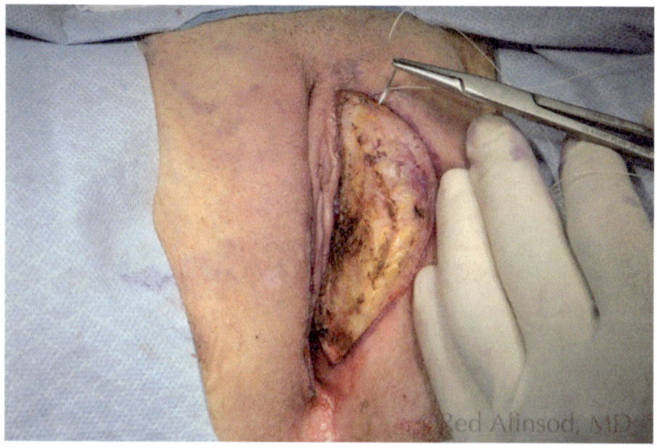

Fig. 2.8 Layered suturing of labia majora

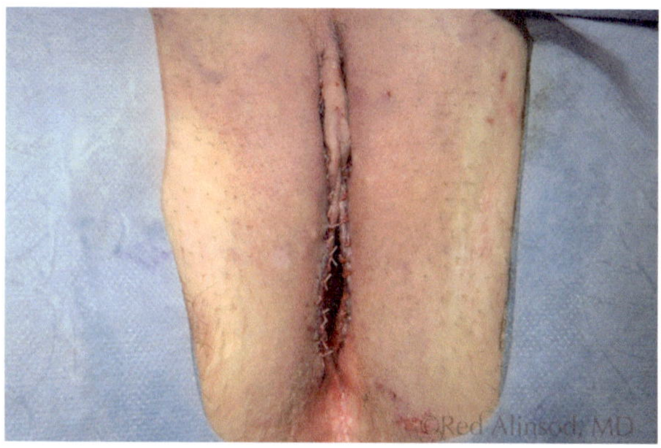

Fig. 2.9 Immediately after labia majoraplasty

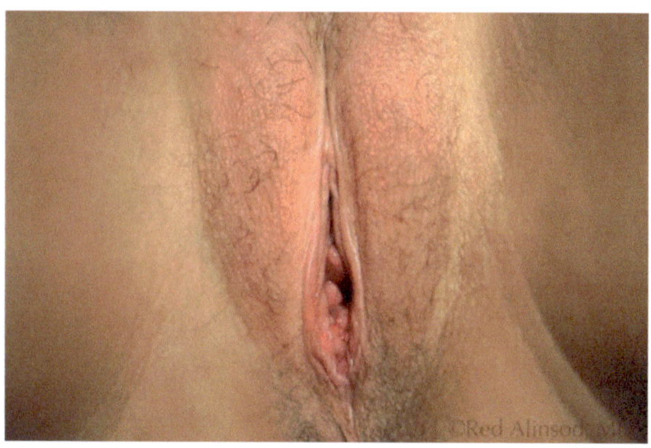

Fig. 2.10 Before

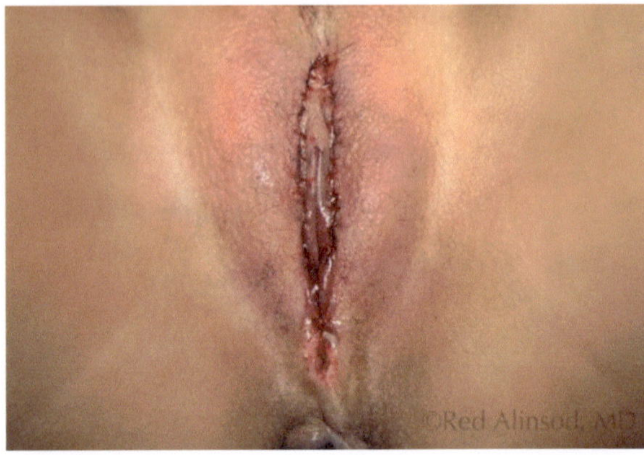

Fig. 2.11 Immediately after

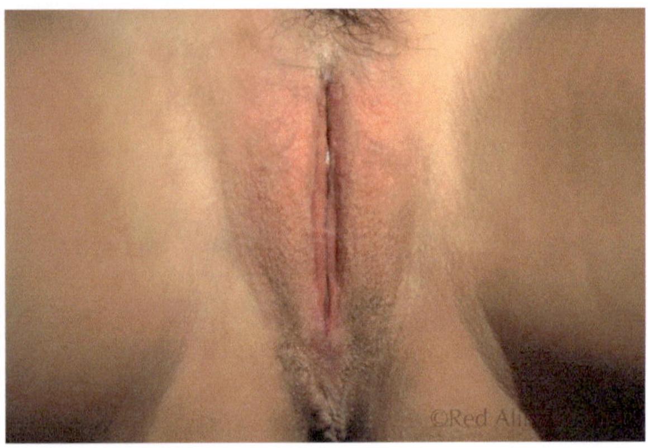

Fig. 2.12 Six weeks after surgery

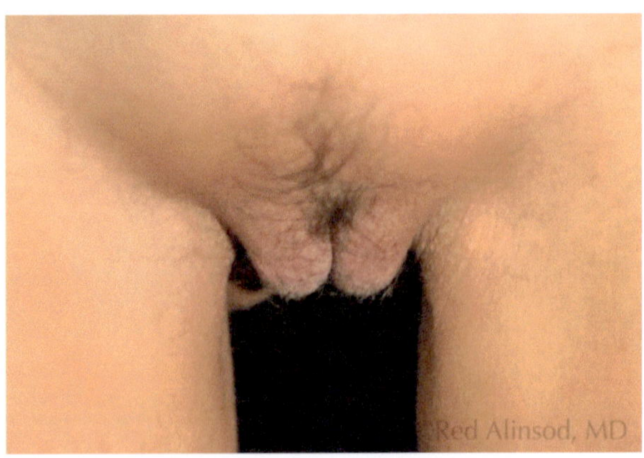

Fig. 2.13 Standing before surgery

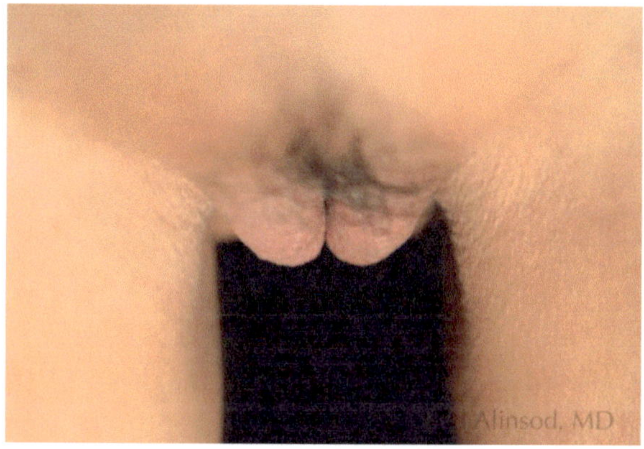

Fig. 2.14 Standing after surgery

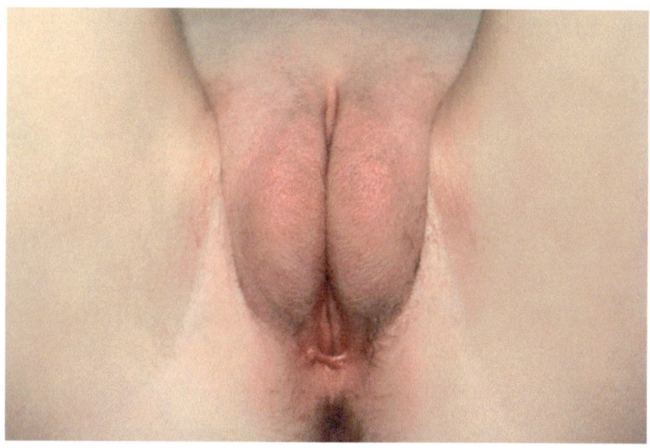

Fig. 2.15 Front before surgery

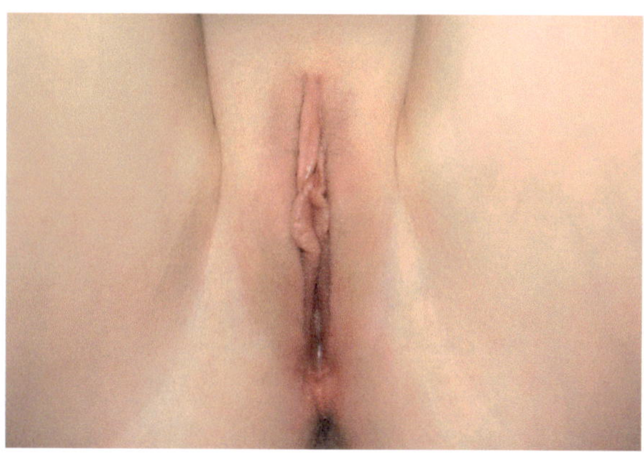

Fig. 2.16 Front after surgery

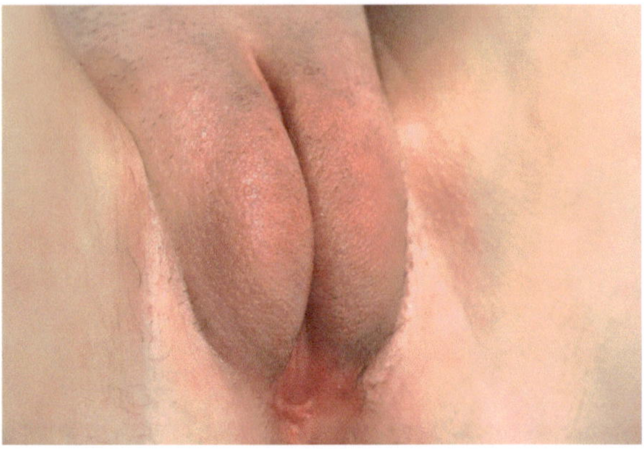

Fig. 2.17 Side before surgery

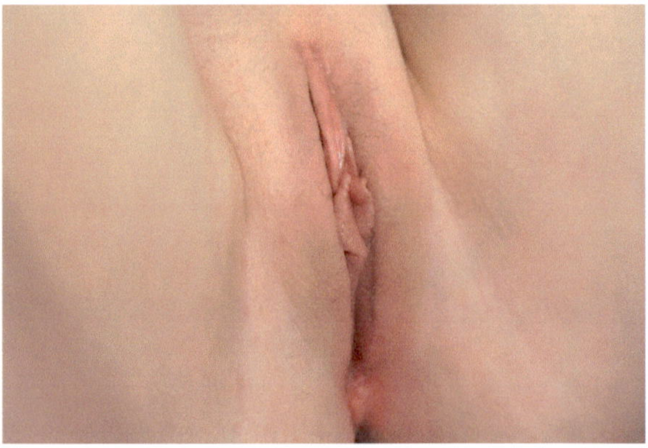

Fig. 2.18 Side after surgery

Chapter 3
Labia Majora Anatomy

Pablo Gonzalez Isaza and Gustavo Parra

The development of the external genitalia in males and females is derived from intermediate mesoderm. It begins in the fourth week when mesenchymal cells from the primitive streak migrate to the cloacal membrane to form a pair of **cloacal folds** [1]. In females, under the influence of estrogens the urogenital and labioscrotal folds are responsible for the development of both labia minora and majora, which arise anteriorly from the mons pubis and fuse posteriorly to form the posterior labial commissure [2]. Labia majora are structures within the vulva, along with mons pubis. Recent findings report labia majora dimensions in average of 79.71 mm SD 15.25 mm [3] (Fig. 3.1).

The vulva is covered by keratinized stratified squamous epithelium, although vestibule is nonkeratinized stratified squamous epithelium. Dermis of the labia majora typically contains an admixture of cutaneous adnexal structures that extend to deeper layers:

Eccrine glands are found in small, circumscribed clusters, and sebaceous glands associated with hair follicles are commonly identified at various levels within the labia majora. These glands contain clear foamy cytoplasm, and apocrine-type glands are secretory cuboidal cells which have more abundant eosinophilic cytoplasm with characteristic apical blebbing [4] (Figs. 3.2 and 3.3).

Innervation of the vulva shares complex somatic territories from iliohypogastric, ilioinguinal, and genitofemoral nerves that supply mons pubis and anterolateral aspects of labia majora to pudendal nerve with its branches inferior rectal and perineal nerve responsible for motor innervation to perineal muscles [5]. Vascular supply to labia majora is derived from femoral artery composed of superficial and deep external branches that supply the mons pubis and anterolateral labia majora, and

P. Gonzalez Isaza (✉)
Obstetrics and Gynecology, Urogynecology Minimally Invasive Surgery,
Hospital Universitario San Jorge, Pereira, Colombia

Soranus Center for Funtional and Regenerative Urogynecology, Pereira, Colombia

G. Parra
Profamilia Clinic, Manizales, Colombia

P. Gonzalez Isaza (ed.), *Aesthetic and Functional Alterations of the Labia Majora*, https://doi.org/10.1007/978-3-031-97405-2_3

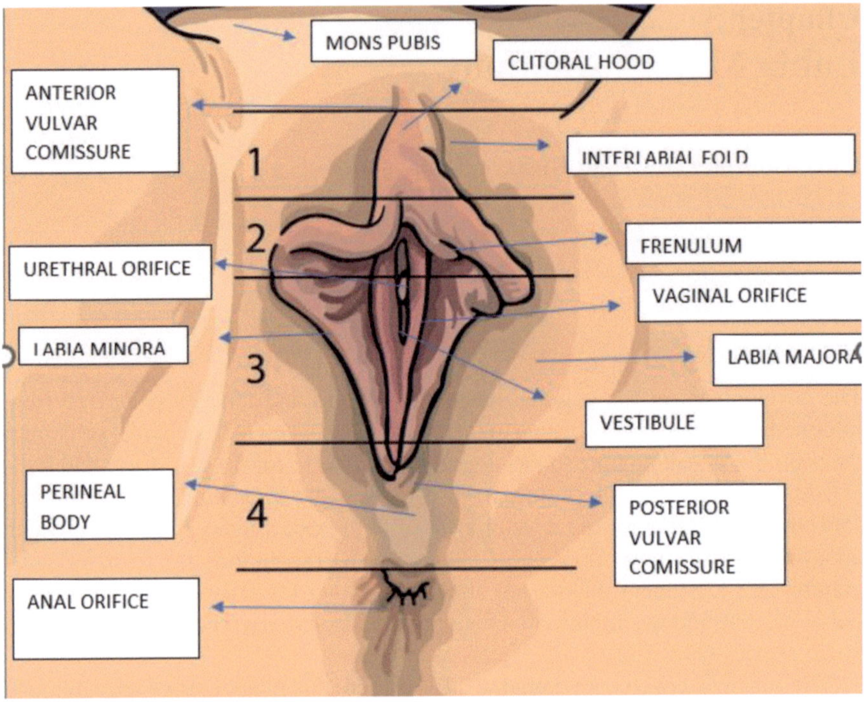

Fig. 3.1 Basic anatomy of the vulva (personal drawing)

also the pudendal artery with its branches perineal posterior and anterior labial arteries is also involved in the vascular supply of labia minora and majora (Fig. 3.4).

Layer by layer there are fascial components that are responsible for functional and aesthetic appearance of the labia majora, campers fascia of the abdominal wall derived from the mesoderm is considered to be the dartos in females, it is a fatty layer mostly composed of areolar tissue that gives structural support to the adipose tissue, Fig. 3A-3B-3C-3D, and it was found in previous examinations of MRI demonstrating a three-dimensional architecture of fibrous septae [6].

A superior attachment is around the xiphoid process and inferiorly the pubic symphysis, were it combines with Scarpa's fascia to form the fatty tissue of the mons pubis and labia majora in females. The function of the fatty layer at the level of labia majora is to absorb mechanical impact from sexual intercourse or sports activities and also to prevent water loss through the skin [7].

Scarpa's fascia also from mesoderm origin is a membranous layer of the anterior abdominal wall, composed of about nine layers; among them, the membranous fascia, thinner than the camper's fascia but more pronounced in females, contains many elastic fibers and loose connective tissue, which offers also mechanical support to the labia majora [7].

Below the fascial components a subcutaneous fat sac is present and bulbospongiosus muscle that attaches caudally to the perineal body, as a deeper

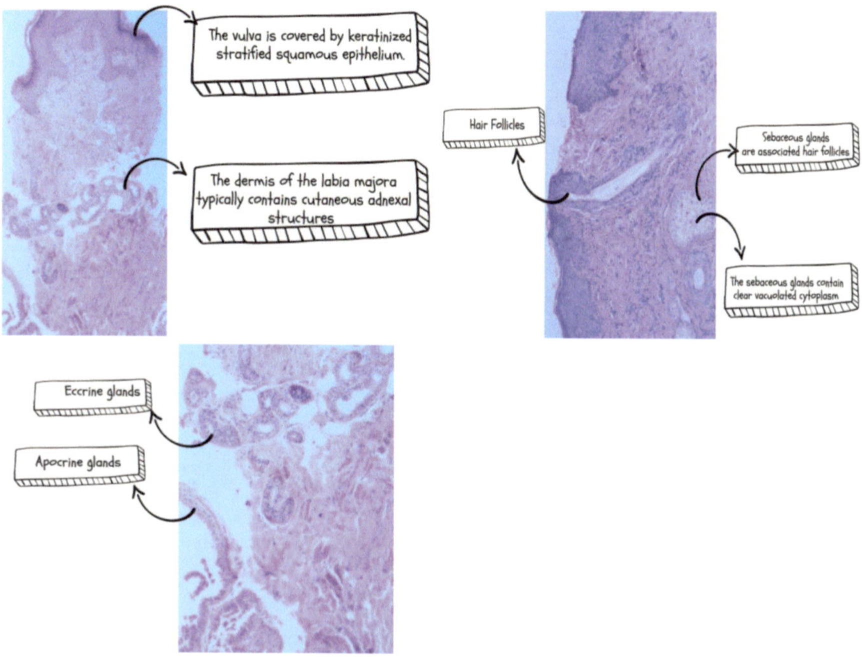

Fig. 3.2 Hematoxylin–eosin stain labia majora histology. Pathology Department. Compensar Bogota Colombia

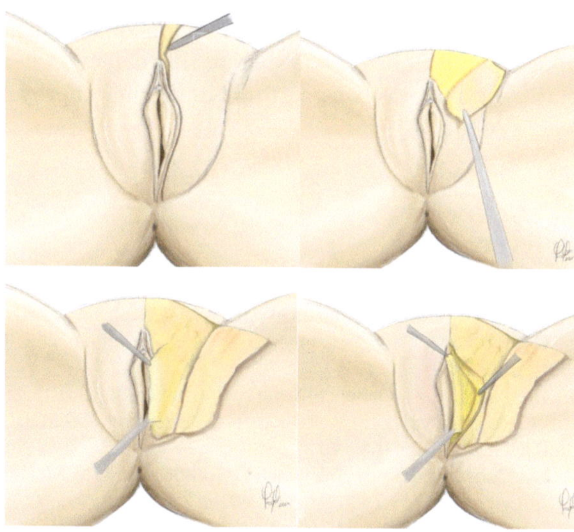

Fig. 3.3 (**a**) Pubic fat. (**b**) Pubic fat extension. (**c**) Superficial fascia. (**d**) Deep fat labial corpus. Layer by layer labia majora and mons pubis anatomical aponeurotic and fat planes. (Courtesy: Dr. Gustavo Parra Colombia)

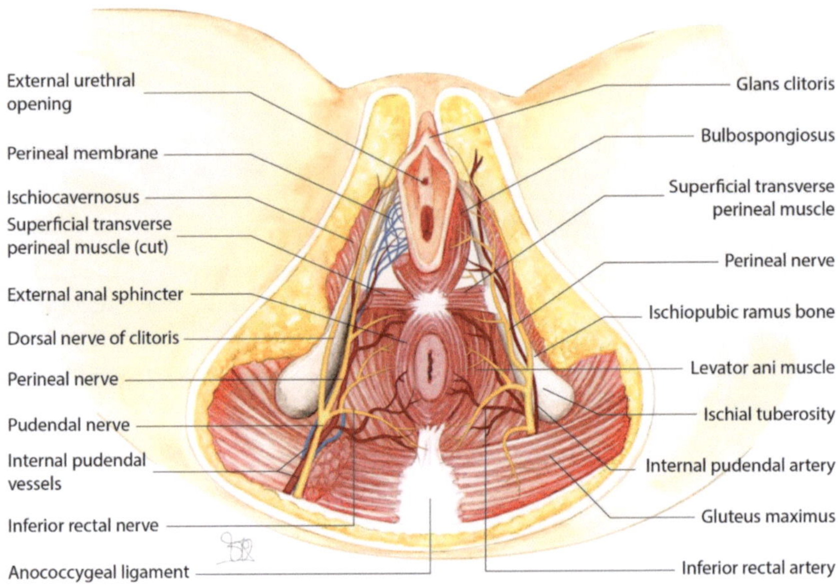

Fig. 3.4 Vascular and nerve supply of labia minora and majora. Elisa Guisantes, Vitoria, Barcelona, Spain

structure the vestibular bulb (erectile body of labia majora) and muscular components (adductor longus, gracilis, adductor magnus, adductor brevis, obturator externus, and obturator internus).Ostrensky et al. described a new anatomical structure identified in fresh cadavers related to subcutaneous fat sac and its relationship with Colles fascia site-specific defects, when identified correctly labiaplasty or labiopexy was performed offering improvement to aesthetic concerns from patients [8].

References

1. Sadler TW. Langman's medical embryology. 12th ed. Philadelphia: Wolters Kluwer; 2012.
2. Carlson BM. Human embryology and developmental biology. 4th ed. Philadelphia: Mosby; 2009.
3. Kreklau A, Vaz I, Oehme F, Strub F, Brechb€uhl R, Christmann C, G€unthert A. Measurements of a 'normal vulva' in women aged 15–84: a cross-sectional prospective single-Centre study. BJOG. 2018;125:1656–61.
4. Lindberg MR, Lamps LW, Quick CM, McKenney JK, McHugh JB. Normal histology. 2nd ed. Elsevier Science Health Science; 2017.
5. Drake RL, Vogl AW, Mitchell AWM. Gray's anatomy for students. 2nd ed. Philadelphia: Churchill Livingstone; 2010.

6. MacKay MD, Mudreac A, Varacallo M. Anatomy, abdomen and pelvis, camper fascia. [updated 2022 Aug 8]. In: Stat pearls [internet]. Treasure Island (FL): Stat Pearls Publishing; 2022. Available from: https://www.ncbi.nlm.nih.gov/books/NBK482246/.
7. Joshi R, Duong H. Anatomy, abdomen and pelvis, Scarpa fascia. [updated 2022 Aug 8]. In: Stat pearls [internet]. Treasure Island (FL): Stat Pearls Publishing; 2022. Available from: https://www.ncbi.nlm.nih.gov/books/NBK553137/.
8. Ostrzenski A, Krajewski P, Davis K. Anatomy and histology of the newly discovered adipose sac structure within the labia majora: international original research. Arch Gynecol Obstet. 2016;294(3):549–54. https://doi.org/10.1007/s00404-016-4052-7. Epub 2016 Apr 11. PMID: 27067433.

Chapter 4
Labia Majora Classifications

Pablo Gonzalez Isaza

Fasola et al. proposed a standardized classification in three stages for labia majora related to the degree of hypotrophy [1], appearance of the skin, and subcutaneous structures and functional complaints from patients.

The aesthetic desires by women regarding the labia majora were categorized in 2022 in the International Journal of Urogynecology where Stage 0 desires no alteration, Stage I desires augmentation, and Stage II desires reduction with added suffixes for laxity (L) and asymmetry (A). This system is very useful because it addresses aesthetic and functional concerns from patients [2].

Ostrensky et al. described a new anatomical structure identified in fresh cadavers related to subcutaneous fat sac and its relationship with Colles fascia site-specific defects, when identified correctly labiaplasty or labiopexy was performed offering improvement to aesthetic concerns from patients [3, 4].

Due to the lack of standardization, guidelines, and nomenclature related to labia majora aesthetic and functional concerns, we aimed to propose a structured classification that guides female cosmetic genital surgeons to determine the most appropriate treatments for different labia majora conditions, such as laxity/loss of tone (related to physiological and mechanical effects, dartos site-specific defects, and fat pad defects), atrophic conditions of the vulva (related to menopause and pharmacological effects), and excess of fat pad (related to weight gain, antiretroviral therapy, metabolic or iatrogenic origin), and each one can generate a variety of functional and esthetic concerns for women.

P. Gonzalez Isaza (✉)
Obstetrics and Gynecology, Urogynecology Minimally Invasive Surgery, Hospital Universitario San Jorge, Pereira, Colombia

Soranus Center for Funtional and Regenerative Urogynecology, Pereira, Colombia

P. Gonzalez Isaza (ed.), *Aesthetic and Functional Alterations of the Labia Majora*, https://doi.org/10.1007/978-3-031-97405-2_4

1. **Cutaneous Hyperlaxity (CHL):** It can be related to aging, chronic friction, waxing, massive weight loss, or after bariatric surgery clinically this part of our classification can be subdivided as shown below.
   - **Mild**: Skin returns to its original position after stretching.
   - **Moderate**: Skin with a saggy appearance slowly returns to a similar position after stretching.
   - **Severe**: Generalized skin laxity, saggy appearance, does not return to its original position after stretching most of the time.
2. **Adipose Hypertrophy (AH):** It is usually related to an excess of fat pad inside labia majora from a metabolic origin and overweight conditions. It can be approached with liposuction, intracavitary RF, or fat pad excision.

   It is important to rule out specific defects of the dartos fascia and fat pad, either clinically by irregular lumps on the surface of the involved labia majora or by ultrasound. The surgical plan generally consists of a fascial plication or a site-specific defect correction that allows closure of the defect.
3. **Cutaneous Adipose Atrophy (CAA)**: Its common causes are hormonal deprivation and lack of response of estrogen receptors responsible for a loss of subcutaneous fat, muscle fiber hypotrophy, and relaxation of connective tissue, and it can be from natural origin or related to oncological treatments, aging, appropriate treatments for these conditions such as fillers with adequate rheological conditions for its use in this area, and autologous fat grafting.
4. **Iatrogenic Conditions (IC):** labia majora deformation secondary to excess of volume injection of autologous fat, hyaluronic acid compounds, or permanent fillers like silicone derivatives. These conditions can be approached with direct skin and fat pad excision.

The following nomenclature is proposed in which a specific letter is assigned to each clinical condition of the labia majora (Table 4.1).

Table 4.1 Different etiological conditions related to aesthetic and functional concerns of labia majora

Cutaneous Hyperlaxity CHL	Adipose Hypertrophy AH	CutaneousAdipose Atrophy CAA	Iatrogenic Conditions IC
Aging Chronic Friction Waxing Weight Loss	Metabolic Overweight Conditions	Menopause Trauma Aging Oncological treatments	Deformation Excess of volume Fillers Fat Silicone derivates

Cutaneous Hyperlaxity (CHL); Adipose Hypertrophy (AH); Cutaneous Adipose Atrophy (CAA); Iatrogenic Conditions (IC)

The dominant location of the defect is then identified and given a specific letter.

Apical (A); Central (C); Perineal (P); Generalized (G)

Its relationship with the fascial components responsible for labia majora tone and elasticity was also identified in a specific letter.

Unilateral (U); Bilateral (B)

References

1. Fasola E, Gazzola R. Labia Majora augmentation with hyaluronic acid filler: technique and results. Aesthet Surg J. 2016;36(10):1155–63. https://doi.org/10.1093/asj/sjw083. Epub 2016 May 30. PMID: 27241363.
2. Developed by the Joint Writing Group of the International Urogynecological Association and the American Urogynecologic Society. Joint report on terminology for cosmetic gynecology. Int Urogynecol J 2022;33(6):1367–1386. doi: https://doi.org/10.1007/s00192-021-050107. Epub 2022 May 23. PMID: 35604421.
3. Ostrzenski A. Labiopexy and Labioplasty for labium Majus rejuvenation in light of a newly discovered anatomic structure. Aesth Plast Surg. 2014;38:554–60.
4. Ostrzenski A, Krajewski P, Davis K. Anatomy and histology of the newly discovered adipose sac structure within the labia majora: international original research. Arch Gynecol Obstet. 2016;294(3):549–54. https://doi.org/10.1007/s00404-016-4052-7. Epub 2016 Apr 11. PMID: 27067433.

Chapter 5
Sonoanatomy of Labia Majora

Enrique Tang-Villanueva and Pablo Gonzalez Isaza

5.1 Introduction

Knowledge of morphological and surgical anatomy is the key to perform percutaneous procedures; in interventional radiology and minimally invasive surgery, it is not possible to prepare or perform procedures without ultrasound-guided visualization, which is the main tool in the evaluation of anatomy to make decisions, choose a therapeutic plan, and select the appropriate materials for each patient and/or procedure. Currently, high-resolution and very high-resolution ultrasound is a portable, accessible, and easy-to-use tool. Any individual with several hours of training can acquire skills to use the ultrasound; an example is the NASA ADUM project [1]. The use of the ultrasound improves safety and controls the results of each diagnostic and therapeutic decision. In alterations, functional and aesthetic procedures in the labia majora of the female genitals and soft tissue ultrasound offer important and innovative contributions to define therapeutic plans, injection volumes, and controlled personalized results [2–5].

"**Real-time ultrasound-guided anatomical dissection**" is the proper use of ultrasound in medical practice for all percutaneous and surgical procedures.

The most important uses of ultrasound as a fundamental tool in interventional radiology available for all surgical and percutaneous techniques [6] are:

E. Tang-Villanueva (✉)
Radiologist, MSK and Soft Tissue Interventionist, Pereira, Colombia
e-mail: info@ultrasonolab.com

P. Gonzalez Isaza
Obstetrics and Gynecology, Urogynecology Minimally Invasive Surgery, Hospital Universitario San Jorge, Pereira, Colombia

Soranus Center for Funtional and Regenerative Urogynecology, Pereira, Colombia

P. Gonzalez Isaza (ed.), *Aesthetic and Functional Alterations of the Labia Majora*, https://doi.org/10.1007/978-3-031-97405-2_5

1. **Assess anatomy in real time:** Scan topography to determine surgical history, past injected products, anatomical variants, metabolic changes, and chronic or acute injuries.
2. **Determine the therapeutic window:** Define more precisely how to navigate the water or cannula to the plane or place where we need to perform the procedure with fewer risk zones, possible complications, and navigation space.
3. **Know the anatomical planes:** Measure and control depths, extensions, volumes, and diameters of the topography to be treated.
4. **Plan the procedure safely:** Observe vascular irrigation, nerve innervation, anatomical variants, nodes, collections and lesions, on an anatomy, choosing the materials, dilutions, planes, techniques, and protocols in a personalized way.
5. **Real-time step-by-step guidance of the procedure:** Guide our needle or cannula to our target, keeping the planes safe and risk areas monitored in real time.
6. **Monitoring therapeutic results:** Monitor results in real time during the procedure and in follow-up checks, identifying injuries or possible associated complications.
7. **Resolve complications:** Determine an injury or complication immediately, with the ability to resolve quickly, safely, and in a controlled manner.
8. **Projecting results:** Knowing the true results of the treatment, previous conditions and the in vivo development, controlled by ultrasound, evaluating the anatomy in real time, knowing the evolution, and generating the quantitative and qualitative scientific capacity to improve your techniques, protocols, and selection of materials.

In order to be a good ultrasound operator and acquire skills to operate the device, it is necessary to know at least how the attenuation of ultrasound in the states of matter, solid, liquid, gaseous, and their transitions composes the ultrasound image in echostructures, understanding that ultrasound is attenuated by matter, this matter can be anatomy, a needle, cannula, a product, substance, changes associated with metabolism, physiology, pathophysiology, and results of a procedure, which determines how the image is composed and its interpretation by the operator. An example of this skill in ultrasound training is acquiring ultrasound anatomical awareness [7].

Think for a moment, **how would an acute collection, a hematoma, for example, look in its acute stage?** Indeed, it will be seen as a liquid image; therefore, in its echostructure it would be anechoic. However, we know that the passage of time generates a transition from liquid to solid, and this will depend on pathophysiological processes, generating septa, capsule, and solidification, among others; this transition will generate differences in ultrasound attenuation and differences in composition in the ultrasound image or echostructures.

Morphological anatomy is the key to performing procedures accurately; ultrasound-guided anatomy provides us with high security.

Learning how to use the ultrasound scanner and the concepts or fundamentals of ultrasound and ultrasound instrumentation are becoming more standardized every day, according to the latest consensus published in 2022, on continuing medical education in ultrasound [8].

Acquiring these concepts with **ultrasound anatomical awareness** is the beginning to perform ultrasound-guided procedures with high precision, as well as understanding that ultrasound and its image composition is directly proportional to the frequency of the transducer; in aesthetic gynecology, to evaluate the soft tissues and structures of the labia majora, we will select devices with high frequency or very high frequency, over 12 MHz, which is more accessible in our health system, to evaluate from the skin and its surface planes to no more than 6 cm deep with high-quality image resolution [9–11].

One of the most important concepts for instrumenting the ultrasound is the frequency, a tip to understand it would be "**the higher the frequency, the less depth and higher the image resolution,**" and according to this tip, the more frequency the device has, the higher image quality you will get in the ultrasound that we will do in soft tissues that share the topography of the labia majora of our patient.

According to our definition of ultrasound "**real-time anatomical dissection guided by ultrasound**" to correctly evaluate the genital region, we suggest starting with the evaluation from the mons pubis, observing the surface structure that is most easily recognized: the pubis (Fig. 5.1) in a cross section, evaluating from the anterior cortex to the surface the corresponding anatomical planes, including the pyramidal muscle to the transition with the rectus abdominis, thus, being able to determine the diameters and thickness of each one of them, and in this section we can perform an ultrasound scan toward the cephalad, on the mons pubis, acquiring images of the topography to recognize the areas with more adipose tissue and vascularity, which we can mark using the metrics of the transducer footprint [12].

The manipulation and use of the transducer language is essential for the acquisition of the image in an adequate manner; this skill in the instrumentation of the ultrasound is one of the fundamental concepts for the good evaluation of the anatomy: Rotate, angle, sweep, and compress are the most important maneuvers to identify an image in real time [8, 13]. Using at each moment of the ultrasound anatomical evaluation, the evaluation modes [14] [15], B Mode, Color Doppler Mode, and Power Doppler Mode, give us precise information on anatomical planes, flow direction, and vascular flow of the evaluated topography (Figs. 5.3 and 5.6).

In our second position, we go to the inguinal fold looking for the Mickey Mouse sign (Fig. 5.2) which is the ultrasound image composed of CFA, common femoral artery; CFV, common femoral vein; and SFJ, sapheno-femoral junction. In this visual, we can go through the veins and arteries in their entire length observing the femoral artery, iliac artery, epigastric artery, superficial circumflex iliac artery, and superficial external pudendal artery, which arise from the femoral just below the crural arch in the region of the femoral triangle, similarly to the gracilis muscles, long adductor muscle, pectineus muscle, and internal obturator muscle (Figs. 5.4, 5.5, and 5.6).

We perform a scan toward the genital region observing the transition of the muscles of the femoral triangle toward the urogenital triangle, observing the topographic planes of the labia majora, identifying the ischiocavernosus, bulbospongiosus, and superficial transverse muscles of the perineum, with the anterior cortex of the

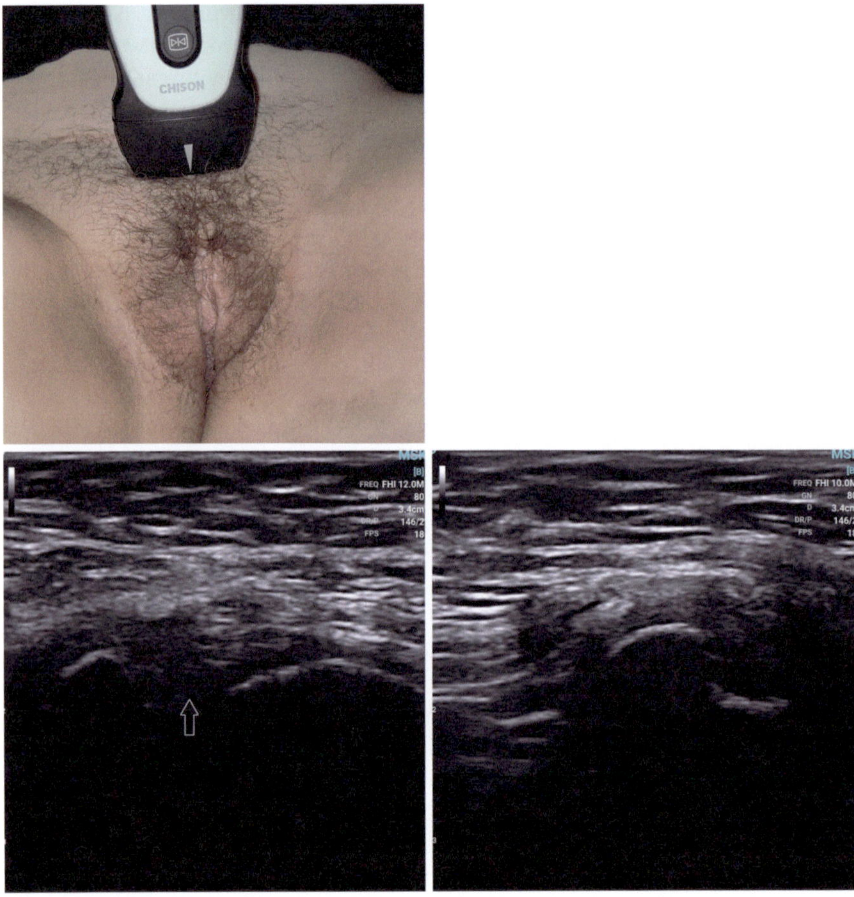

Fig. 5.1 Sonoeye P1 Linear Transducer by Chison, up to 14 MHz, selected for this image at 10 MHz, positioned over the pubis, showing the ultrasound anatomy, cortical line of the pubis, and soft tissue planes in both longitudinal and transverse sections, with a depth of 3.5 cm observed

ischium being our most inferior point of the ultrasound anatomical repair (Figs. 5.7 and 5.8).

Evaluating Camper's fascia and its transition to Colles' fascia [16] is the most intuitive way to detail the ultrasound anatomical planes with great precision, Colles' fascia being the one that allows us to determine the superficial plane in percutaneous procedures, a safe area with subcutaneous cellular tissue over the labia majora [17] (Fig. 5.9).

Bartholin's glands are limited by the lower plane of the labia majora, making the ultrasound scan limited by the vaginal canal in the internal plane, until visualizing the Bartholin gland, observing transition planes in its echostructures, normal and possible pathological findings [18] (Fig. 5.10).

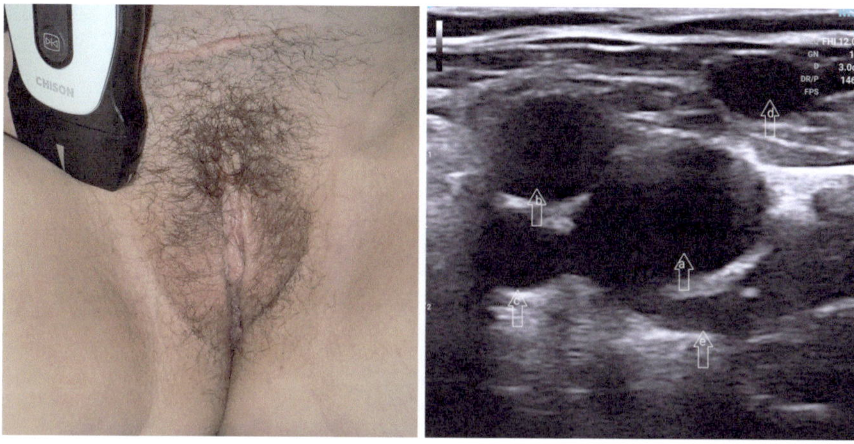

Fig. 5.2 Sonoeye P1 Linear Transducer by Chison, up to 14 MHz, selected at 10 MHz in the right inguinal fold, demonstrating the "Mickey Mouse" sign: (**a**) Common Femoral Vein, (**b**) Common Femoral Artery, (**c**) Femoral Artery, (**d**) Magna Saphenous Vein, and (**e**) Deep Femoral Vein. We observed the surrounding soft tissues

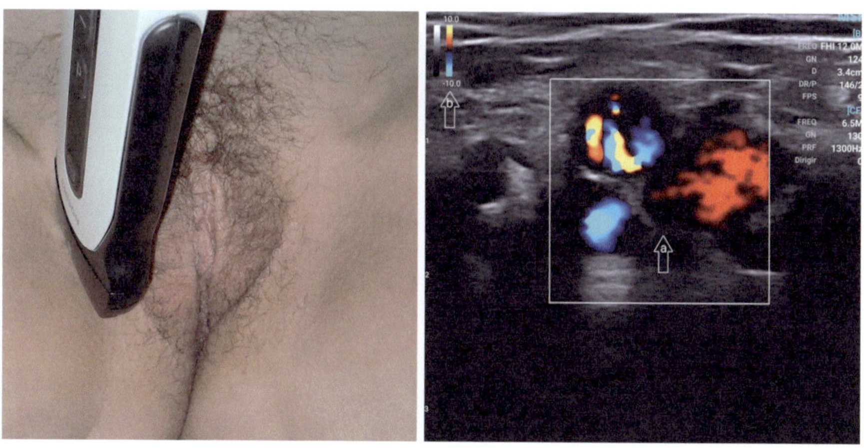

Fig. 5.3 Sonoeye P1 Linear Transducer by Chison, up to 14 MHz, selected at 10 MHz in the right inguinal fold with slight angulation and rotation according to the transducer manipulation. The direction of vascular flow obtained using Color Doppler mode is observed; the blue color suggests that the flow is deeper, while the red color indicates a more superficial flow

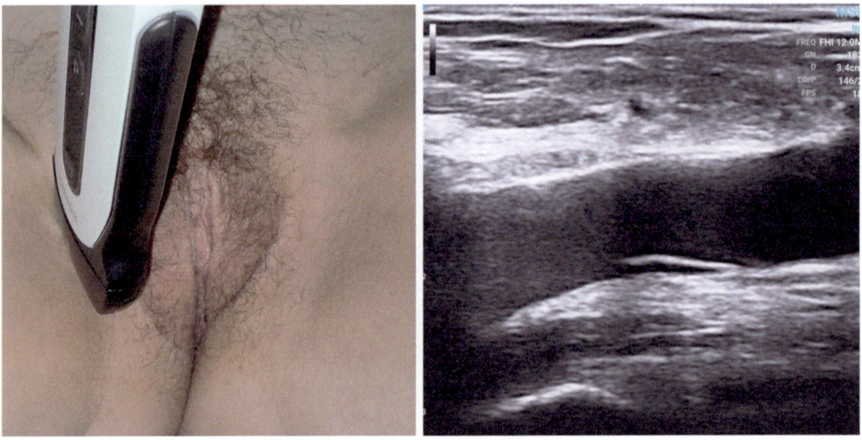

Fig. 5.4 Sonoeye P1 Linear Transducer by Chison, up to 14 MHz, selected at 12 MHz in the right inguinal fold with slight angulation and rotation according to the transducer's orientation. The Great Saphenous Vein is observed in longitudinal view, with the valves inside in the process of opening

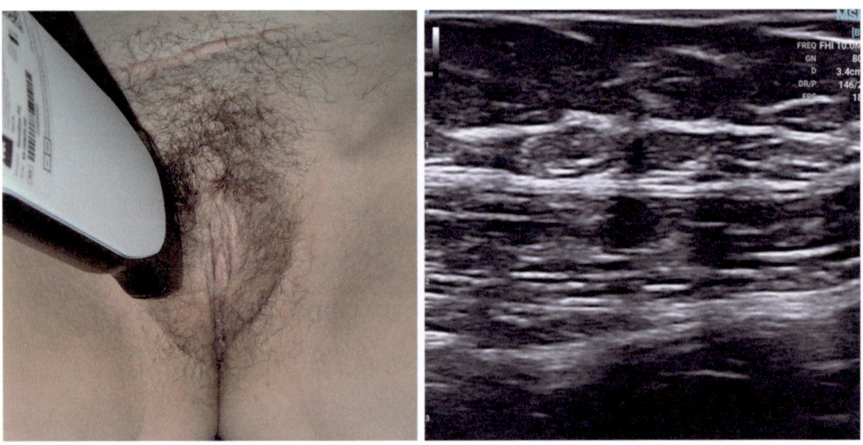

Fig. 5.5 Sonoeye P1 Linear Transducer by Chison, up to 14 MHz, selected at 10 MHz, positioned over the vulvar transition, observing from superficial to deep: skin, subcutaneous cellular tissue without compression, superficial fascia (Colles), and bulbospongiosus muscle

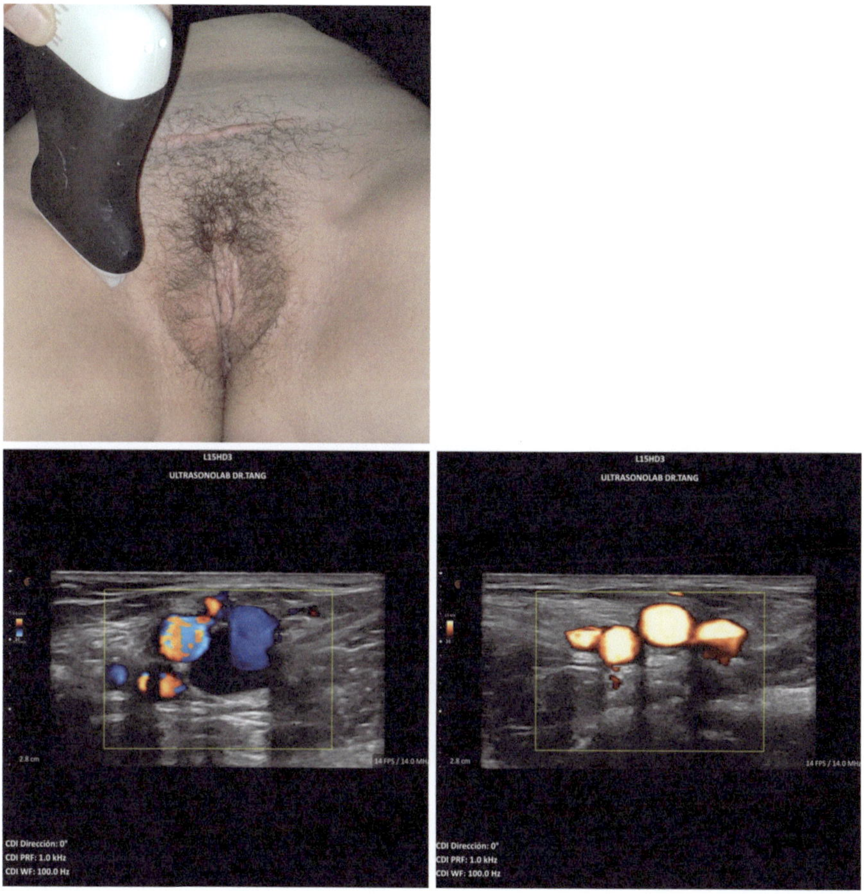

Fig. 5.6 (1) Clarius L15 Linear Transducer, up to 15 MHz, selected at 14 MHz, positioned in the inguinal fold, observed during ultrasound scanning with angulation, demonstrating the "Mickey Mouse" sign with Color Doppler mode confirming the direction of flow. (2) The Power Doppler mode, confirming vascular flow

Vascular flow and flow direction are of great importance for planning a percutaneous procedure. Observing the depth in the plane, anteroposterior diameter, location, and extension on the surface gives us the possibility of preventing possible injuries or complications, such as obstruction or obliteration, mainly in injections with hyaluronic acid. Knowing the vascular anatomy is essential, and the use of ultrasound makes it easier for us to determine with precision and in a personalized way [19] (Fig. 5.6).

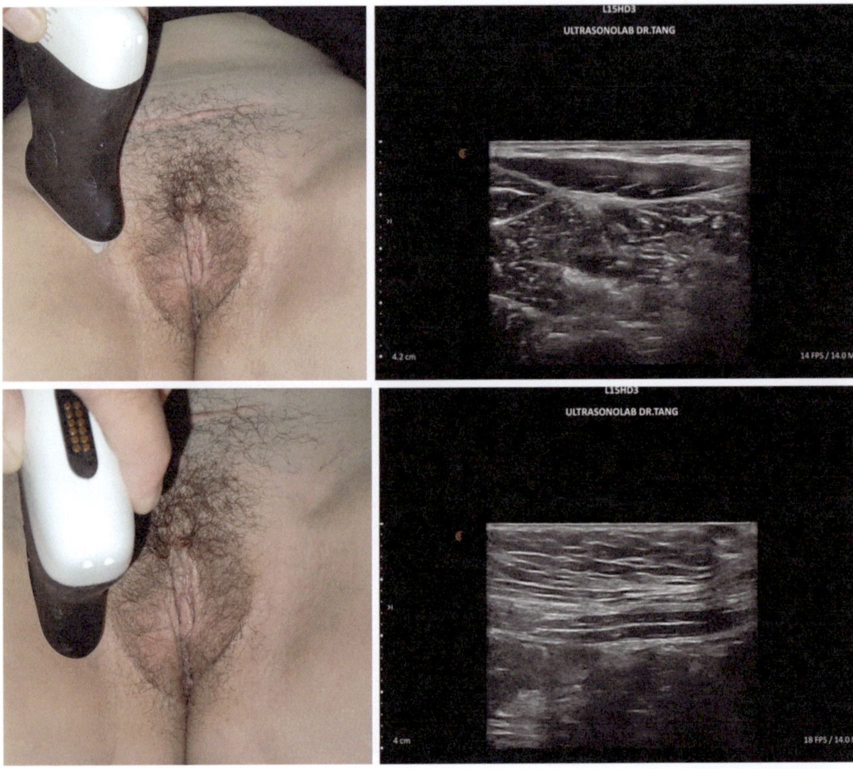

Figs. 5.7 and 5.8 Clarius L15 Linear Transducer, up to 15 MHz, selected at 14 MHz, positioned in the inguinal fold, performing a transition during ultrasound scanning with rotation and angulation toward the vulva, observing Fig. 5.7. Skin, Subcutaneous Cellular Tissue, Superficial Fascia, Gracilis Muscle, Adductor Magnus, Adductor Longus, and Femur. Figure 5.8 Skin, Subcutaneous Cellular Tissue, Superficial Fascia (Colles), Ischiocavernosus Muscle, and Deep Fascia (Perineal Membrane)

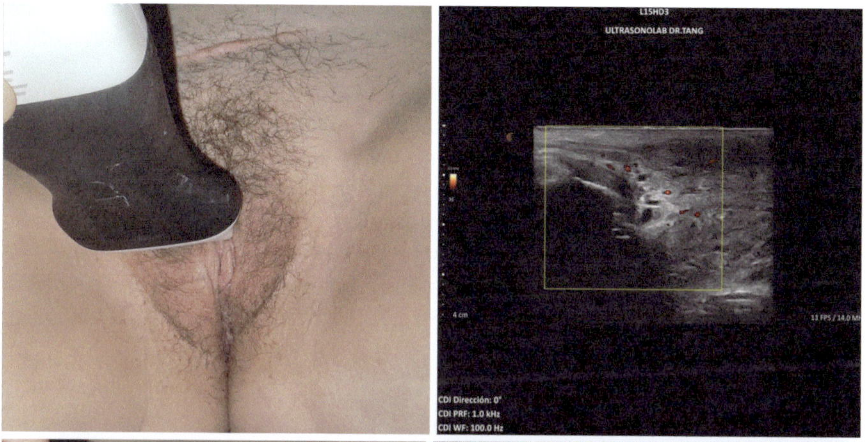

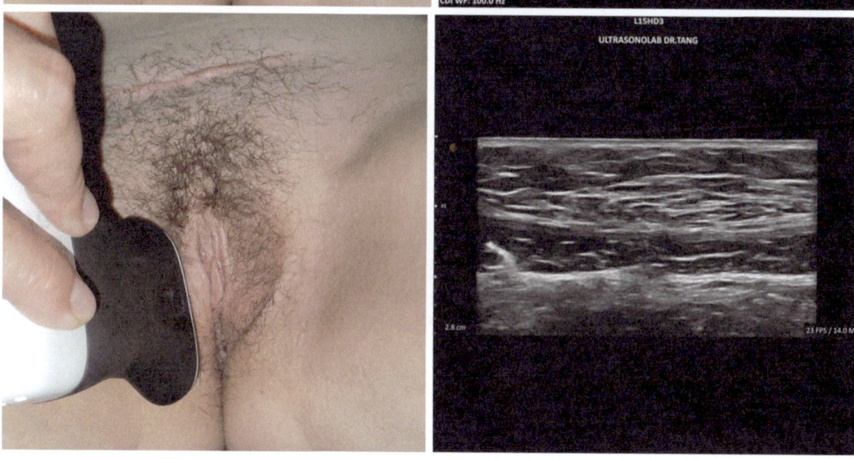

Figs. 5.9 and 5.10 Clarius L15 Linear Transducer, up to 15 MHz, selected at 14 MHz, positioned at the transition of the vulva and over the vulva with longitudinal and transverse rotation of the superficial anatomy, observing in both images: Skin, Subcutaneous Cellular Tissue, Superficial Fascia, Gracilis Muscle, Adductor Magnus, Adductor Longus, and Femur. Figure 5.10 Skin, Subcutaneous Cellular Tissue, Superficial Fascia (Colles), Ischiocavernosus Muscle, Deep Fascia (Perineal Membrane), confirming the direction of vascular flow with Color Doppler mode in Fig. 5.9

5.2 Conclusion

Evaluating the anatomy of the pelvic floor and external genitalia with real-time ultrasound gives us the possibility of accurately and personally determining the procedures in aesthetic and functional gynecology, selecting the materials and constantly monitoring the results.

Understanding the use of ultrasound, its fundamentals, transducer language, and device instrumentation requires training directed by an expert. In a short time, you will be able to add its usefulness to your daily routine. Professionals can quickly acquire the technical skills to become experts, based on ultrasound anatomical awareness.

References

1. chrome-extension://efaidnbmnnnibpcajpcglclefindmkaj/. https://www.nasa.gov/wp-content/uploads/2013/11/issrdc_2012-06-26-1000_melton2012.pdf
2. Hersant B, Jabbour SN, Warren, Benadiba L, La Padula S, SidAhmed-Mezi M, Meningaud JP. Labia Majora augmentation combined with minimal labia Minora resection: a safe and global approach to the external female genitalia. Ann Plast Surg. 2018;80(4):323–7. https://doi.org/10.1097/SAP.0000000000001435.
3. Ostrzenski A, Krajewski P, Davis K. Anatomy and histology of the newly discovered adipose sac structure within the labia majora: international original research. Arch Gynecol Obstet. 2016;294:549–54. https://doi.org/10.1007/s00404-016-4052-7.
4. Seleem M, Osman OM, Kashmar SG, Lotfy R. Dimensions, ratios, volumes, and weights of the fatty parts of the vulva (Mons pubis and labia Majora). Aesthet Surg J. 2023;43(9):1002–12. https://doi.org/10.1093/asj/sjad106.
5. Migda MS, Migda M, Słapa R, Mlosek RK, Migda B. The use of high-frequency ultrasonography in the assessment of selected female reproductive structures: the vulva, vagina and cervix. J Ultrason. 2019;19(79):261–8. https://doi.org/10.15557/JoU.2019.0039.
6. https://www.elsevier.es/es-revista-radiologia-119-articulo-intervencionismo-guiado-por-ecografia-lo-S0033833810000603
7. https://www.ardms.org/get-certified/spi/
8. Hoppmann RA, Mladenovic J, Melniker L, et al. International consensus conference recommendations on ultrasound education for undergraduate medical students. Ultrasound J. 2022;14(1):31. Published 2022 Jul 27. https://doi.org/10.1186/s13089-022-00279-1.
9. Izzetti R, Vitali S, Aringhieri G, et al. Ultra-high frequency ultrasound, a promising diagnostic technique: review of the literature and single-center experience. Can Assoc Radiol J. 2021;72(3):418–31. https://doi.org/10.1177/0846537120940684.
10. Levy J, Barrett DL, Harris N, Jeong JJ, Yang X, Chen SC. High-frequency ultrasound in clinical dermatology: a review. Ultrasound J. 2021;13(1):24. Published 2021 Apr 20. https://doi.org/10.1186/s13089-021-00222-w.
11. Russo A, Reginelli A, Lacasella GV, Grassi E, Karaboue MAA, Quarto T, Busetto GM, Aliprandi A, Grassi R, Berritto D. Clinical application of ultra-high-frequency ultrasound. J Pers Med. 2022;12(10):1733. https://doi.org/10.3390/jpm12101733. PMID: 36294872; PMCID: PMC9605054.
12. Borowy CS, Mukhdomi T. Sonography physical principles and instrumentation. [updated 2023 mar 20]. In: StatPearls [internet]. Treasure Island (FL): StatPearls Publishing; 2024. Available from : https://www.ncbi.nlm.nih.gov/books/NBK567710/.

13. End B, Prats MI, Minardi J, Sharon M, Bahner DP, Boulger CT. Language of transducer manipulation 2.0: continuing to codify terms for effective teaching. Ultrasound J. 2021;13(1):44. https://doi.org/10.1186/s13089-021-00245-3. PMID: 34709487; PMCID: PMC8555041.
14. Zander D, Hüske S, Hoffmann B, Cui XW, Dong Y, Lim A, Jenssen C, Löwe A, Koch JBH, Dietrich CF. Ultrasound image optimization (" Knobology "): B- mode. Ultrasound Int Open. 2020;6(1):E14–24. https://doi.org/10.1055/a-1223-1134. Epub 2020 Aug 31. PMID: 32885137; PMCID: PMC7458857.
15. Meola M, Ibeas J, Lasalle G, Petrucci I. Basics for performing a high-quality color Doppler sonography of the vascular access. J Vasc Access. 2021;22(1_suppl):18–31. https://doi.org/10.1177/11297298211018060. Epub 2021 Jul 28. PMID: 34320855; PMCID: PMC8607315.
16. Joshi R, Duong H. Anatomy, abdomen and pelvis, Scarpa fascia. [updated 2023 Aug 7]. In: StatPearls [internet]. Treasure Island (FL): StatPearls Publishing; 2024. Available from : https://www.ncbi.nlm.nih.gov/books/NBK553137/.
17. Roch M, Gaudreault N, Cyr MP, Venne G, Bureau NJ, Morin M. The female pelvic floor fascia anatomy: a systematic search and review. Life (Basel). 2021;11(9):900. https://doi.org/10.3390/life11090900. PMID: 34575049; PMCID: PMC8467746.
18. Cheung VYT. Ultrasonography of benign vulvar injuries. Ultrasonography. 2018;37(4):355–60. https://doi.org/10.14366/usg.18001. Epub 2018 Feb 13. PMID: 29575850; PMCID: PMC6177693
19. Lee H, Yap YL, Low JJ, Lim J. Labia Majora Share. Arch Plast Surg. 2017;44(1):80–4. https://doi.org/10.5999/aps.2017.44.1.80. Epub 2017 Jan 20. PMID: 28194353; PMCID: PMC5300930.

Chapter 6
Labia Majora Labiaplasty Surgical Techniques

Pablo Gonzalez Isaza

From the surgical point of view, there is always a need to consider this option for certain skin laxity conditions, especially after massive weight loss. There are few described techniques inside the scientific literature; most of them involve mainly skin and subcutaneous tissue resection leaving hidden scars inside anatomical landmarks, such as interlabial and crural folds [1, 2].

The amount of skin to be resected is usually calculated with a pinch test, which allows surgeons to be conservative and avoid over resection [3] (Fig. 6.1).

Inside our center, we consider it very important to have hidden and aesthetic scars, which is why we always prefer to perform the technique leaving the scar inside the interlabial fold (Fig. 6.2a–d).

Hunter in 2015 described his technique with more noticeable scars outside the interlabial fold [4] (Fig. 6.3).

When the surgeon faces both labia majora and minora alterations, there is a need to perform what we consider a combined labiaplasty, and there are no standard steps to perform the procedure, but as a general rule, the experience of the surgeon is what matters at the moment of surgery. Miklos and Moore published a case report of combined labiaplasty in a 36-year-old women in 2011; in this case linear labia minora labiaplasty and labia majora labiaplasty with hidden scars were performed with a very good aesthetic surgical outcome [5] (Fig. 6.4).

A recent report from Goodman describes the combination of labia majora and labia minora plasty, at the moment of cutting labia minora "the wing technique"; the

Supplementary Information The online version contains supplementary material available at https://doi.org/10.1007/978-3-031-97405-2_6.

P. Gonzalez Isaza (✉)
Obstetrics and Gynecology, Urogynecology Minimally Invasive Surgery,
Hospital Universitario San Jorge, Pereira, Colombia

Soranus Center for Funtional and Regenerative Urogynecology, Pereira, Colombia

P. Gonzalez Isaza (ed.), *Aesthetic and Functional Alterations of the Labia Majora*, https://doi.org/10.1007/978-3-031-97405-2_6

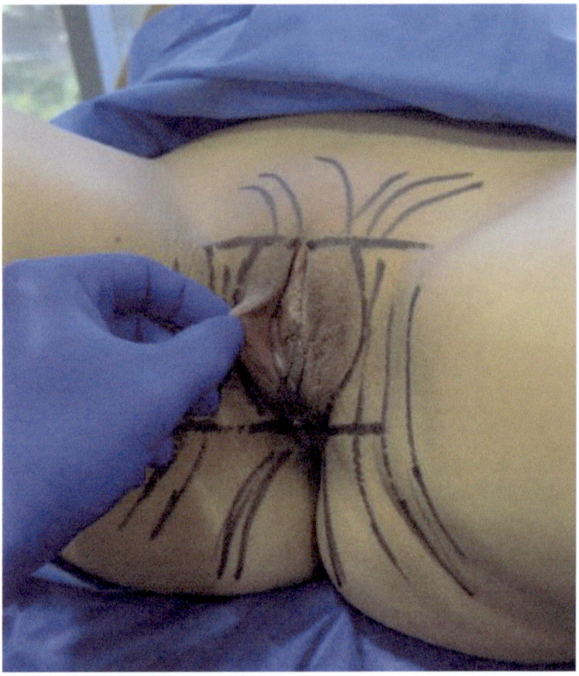

Fig. 6.1 Pinch test to calculate the amount of skin to be excised

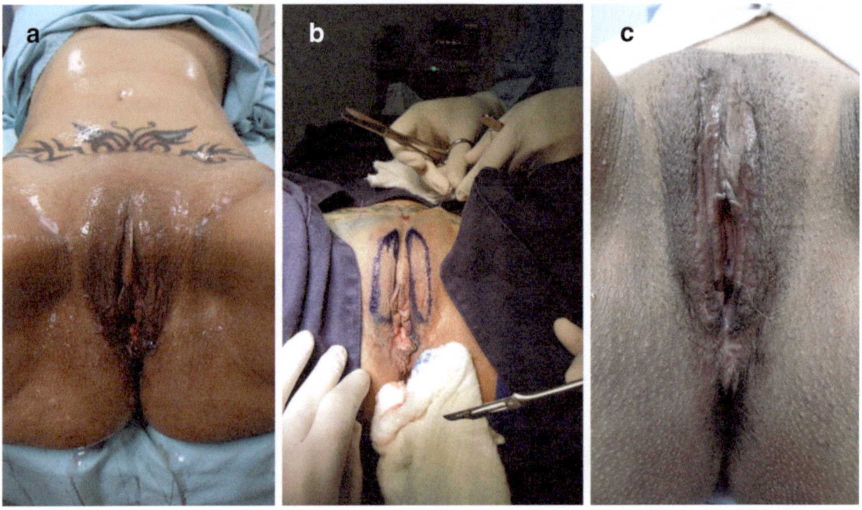

Fig. 6.2 (**a**) Pre-op (**b**) Interlabial fold margins. (**c**) One-month post-op

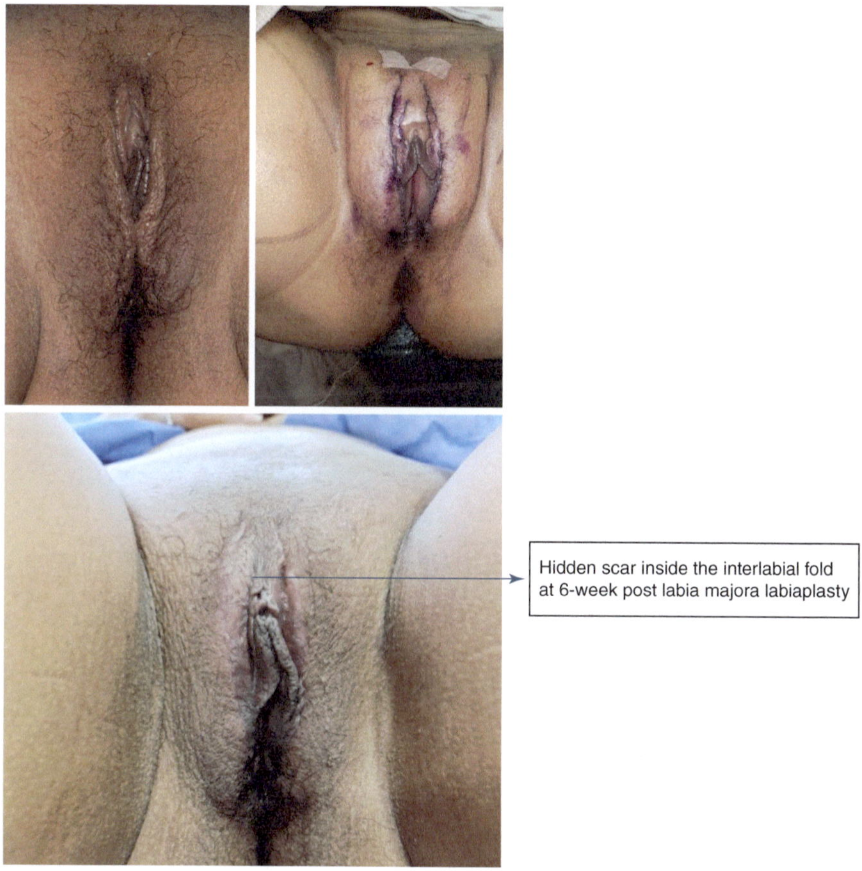

Fig. 6.3 Labia majoraplasty

surgical line is extended to the interlabial fold, involving labia majora skin, improving laxity but unfortunately leaving noticeable scars [6].

Ostrensky et al. described a new anatomical structure identified in fresh cadavers related to subcutaneous fat sac and its relationship with Colles fascia site-specific defects, when identified correctly labiaplasty or labiopexy was performed offering improvement to aesthetic concerns from patients [7].

We have very detailed algorithms of treatment for surgical indications of labia majora; it involves patient desires and surgical possibilities (Table 6.1).

As a first step we evaluate patient expectations regarding labia majora aesthetic goals, and sometimes patients who perform competitive sports, especially those riding bicycle or spinning, prefer to have a flat configuration of labia majora. In this case we choose surgical removal of excess skin, some patients in contrast besides skin resection, and they also want to add some volume to labia majora. For this situation we perform a skin resection, preserving the dartos fascia, and add either autologous fat grafting or fillers (Figs. 6.3, 6.4, 6.5, and 6.6); Video 6.1).

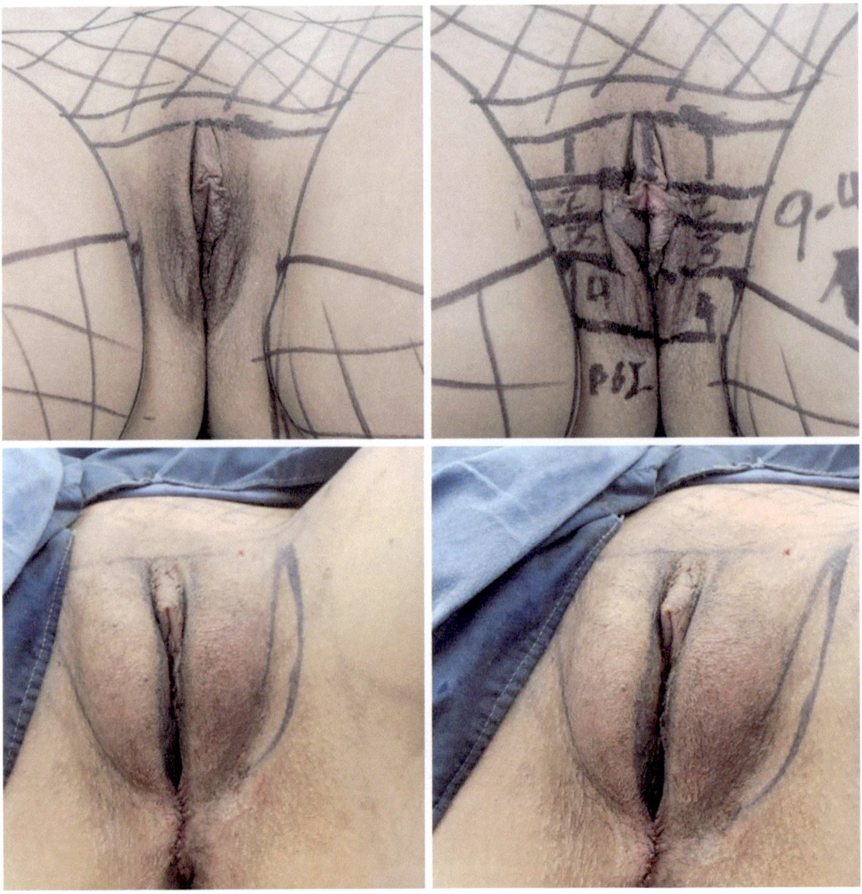

Fig. 6.4 Combined labia minora plasty and labia majora autologous fat grafting

Table. 6.1 Algorithmic approach for labia majora aesthetic and functional indications

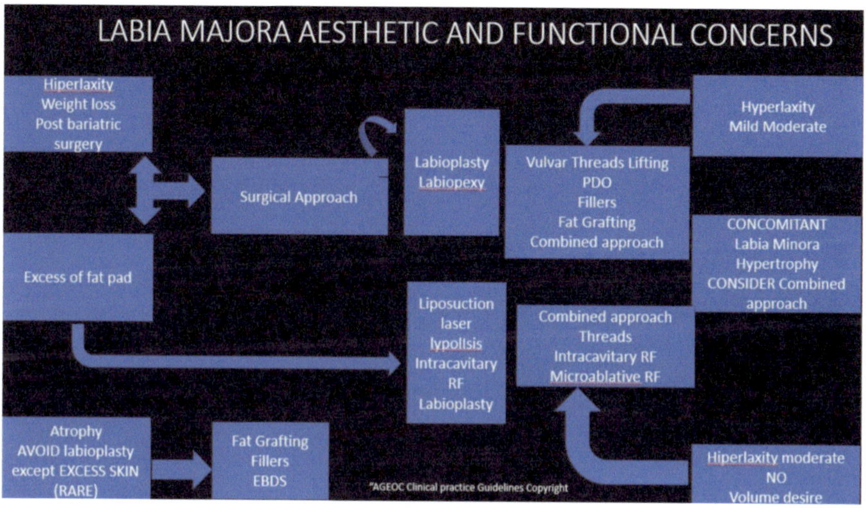

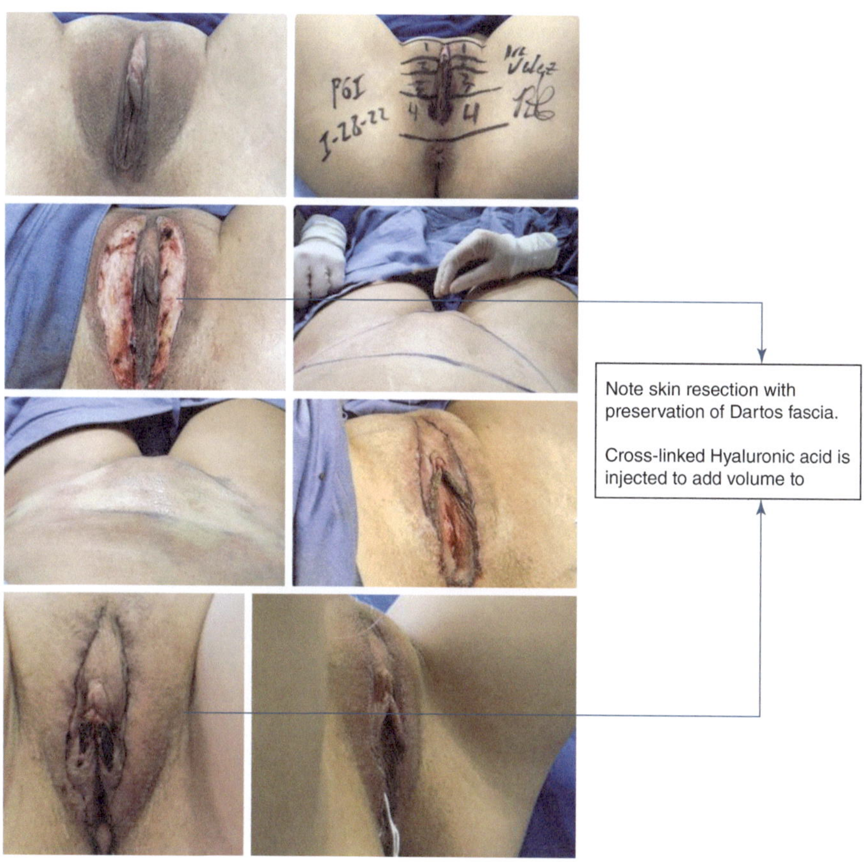

Fig. 6.5 Labia majoraplasty dartos fascia preservation and cross-linked hyaluronic acid injection

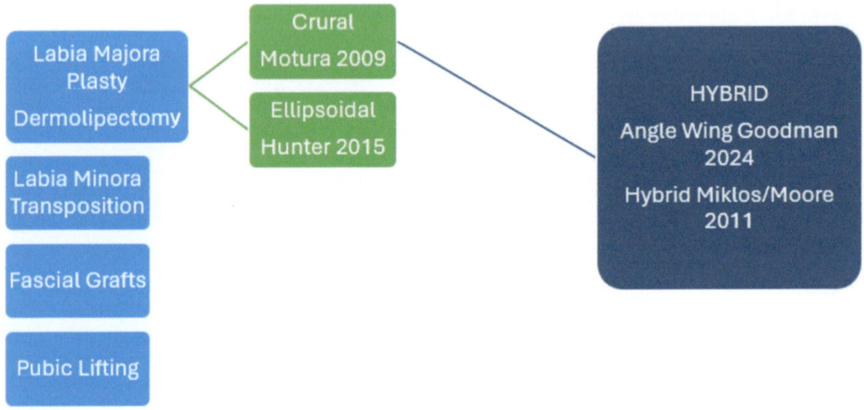

Fig. 6.6 Techniques for surgical management of labia majora aesthetic and functional alterations

References

1. Alter GJ. Pubic contouring after massive weight loss in men and women: correction of hidden penis, Mons ptosis, and labia majora enlargement. Plast Reconstr Surg. 2012;130(4):936–47. https://doi.org/10.1097/PRS.0b013e318262f57d.
2. Mottura AA. Labia majora hypertrophy. Aesth Plast Surg. 2009;33(6):859–63. https://doi.org/10.1007/s00266-008-9260-5.
3. Saheb-Al-Zamani M. Labia Majora reduction (Majoraplasty). Clin Plast Surg. 2022;49(4):489–94. https://doi.org/10.1016/j.cps.2022.06.010.
4. Hunter JG. Labia Minora, labia Majora, and clitoral Hood alteration: experience-based recommendations. Aesthet Surg J. 2016;36(1):71–9. https://doi.org/10.1093/asj/sjv092. Epub 2015 Oct 24
5. Miklos JR, Moore RD. Simultaneous labia minora and majora reduction: a case report. J Minim Invasive Gynecol. 2011;18(3):378–80. https://doi.org/10.1016/j.jmig.2010.12.013.
6. Goodman MP. The "angel-wing" combined labia Minoraplasty/Majoraplasty. Am J Cosmet Surg. 2024;0(0) https://doi.org/10.1177/07488068241243263.
7. Ostrzenski A, Krajewski P, Davis K. Anatomy and histology of the newly discovered adipose sac structure within the labia majora: international original research. Arch Gynecol Obstet. 2016;294(3):549–54. https://doi.org/10.1007/s00404-016-4052-7. Epub 2016 Apr 11

Chapter 7
Indications/Contraindications for Labia Majora Labiaplasty

Diana Lorena Vélez Rizo

Labiaplasty of the labia majora is a highly satisfactory and safe surgical procedure that seeks to restore a youthful appearance to said structure: fillers in the anterior third and narrow fillers in the lower third.

When the woman is standing, the labia majora are almost in the midline and form the anterior commissure, and they are responsible for protecting the vaginal introitus and the labia minora throughout their extension [1, 2].

The labia majora are affected, as well as other areas of the body, by aging, multiparity, gravity, loss of collagen, fat padding, and skin quality [3].

Statistically, the most common procedures performed on the labia majora include augmentation (36.95%), reduction (29%), and mons pubis plasty (26.48%) and are frequently indicated when there is no response to nonsurgical procedures or the defect of the labia majora merits it according to its classification as a severe compromise of tone and laxity that cannot be improved with noninvasive procedures [4–6].

D. L. V. Rizo (✉)
Gynecologist and Obstetrician Universidad de la Sabana, Cundinamarca, Colombia

Colposcopy and Cervical Pathology Universidad Nacional de, Bogotá, Colombia

Laser and Gynecologic Functional Aesthetic Surgery AGEOC Association of Colombian Aesthetic Gynecologists, Bogotá, Colombia

Laser applications in gynecology Universidad Nacional de, Bogotá, Colombia

Master in Clinical Sexology, University of Valencia, Valencia, Spain

Urological and Reconstructive Gynecology of the Pelvic Floor National University of Colombia, Bogotá, Colombia

Gynecologist in Dr. Diana Velez Rizo Advanced Gynecology, Fundación Cardioinfantil and Clínica de la Mujer, Bogotá, Colombia

P. Gonzalez Isaza (ed.), *Aesthetic and Functional Alterations of the Labia Majora*, https://doi.org/10.1007/978-3-031-97405-2_7

The initial guidelines are:

1. Define what are the patient's complaint and her clear expectations about the procedure: What is she looking for? Big, plump lips or, on the contrary, toned lips without volume or sagging? This first step helps us find the most appropriate surgical procedure proposal [1].
2. A complete physical examination in conjunction with the patient that defines according to the dimension, proportion, weight, and volume not only of the labia majora but also of the Mons Venus, additionally considering the body mass index (BMI), in addition to an adequate photographic record standing and in lithotomy position from the front and sides [1, 7, 8].
3. Consider surgical management: Labiaplasty of the labia majora with volume reduction or fat lipotransfer with or without compromising skin [1].

Indications:

- Excess skin of the labia majora with ptosis and loss of tone: Patients frequently indicate difficulty with wearing tight clothing and notoriety with their use.
- Difficulty with penetration due to excess tissue.
- Interference with cleanliness and hygiene.
- Mons Venus ptosis.
- Protrusion and/or elongation of the interlabial fold.
- Concomitant presence of hypertrophy of the labia minora, since when the labia majora are intervened they can increase their notoriety
- History of excessive weight loss [1]
- Patient with deformity secondary to previous surgeries or resection of vulvar pathologies such as Bowen's disease or Lichen sclerosus and atrophicus, among others [9].
- Resection of vertical anatomical variants of the interlabial fold (Fig. 7.1).
- HIV disease, the chronic use of some antiretrovirals (Atazanavir, Darunavir, Fosamprenavir, Ritonavir, Tipranavir, Zidovudine (AZT), and Stavudine), has

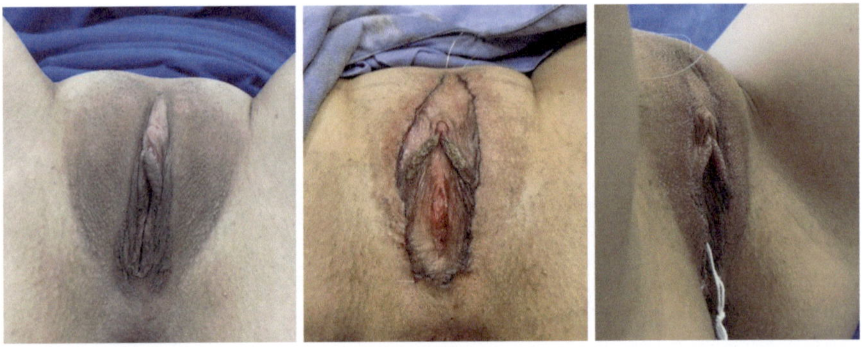

Fig. 7.1 Laxity of the labia majora with vertical anatomical variants that compromise the interlabial fold. Patient taken to Labiaplasty for labia majora reduction and resection of variants in the same incision

been related to lipodystrophy already described in the literature. At the genital level, different symptoms have been reported, ranging from severe hypertrophy of the labia majora and asymmetric loss of their volume, which can only be corrected with surgical management after changing antiretroviral therapy [10].

To keep in mind how much tissue to safely remove, planning and marking must be carried out in the lithotomy position with maximum abduction of the legs, verifying that the interlabial fold area is not tight [1].

7.1 Lipotransfer of Labias Major

In cases that seek to both increase and recover the volume of the tissue of the labia majora, lipotransfer of fat from the lower third of the abdomen or middle face of the thighs not only seeks a more youthful appearance of the lips but is also an excellent tool in reconstructive surgery of the labia minora, mainly when amputations have occurred before and protection of the vulvar midline structures and vaginal introitus is required (Fig. 7.2).

The application of autologous macrofat-type tissue behind the dartos allows an effective and lasting increase in volume taking into account that approximately 30% of the fatty tissue applied can be absorbed in the first postoperative months [1].

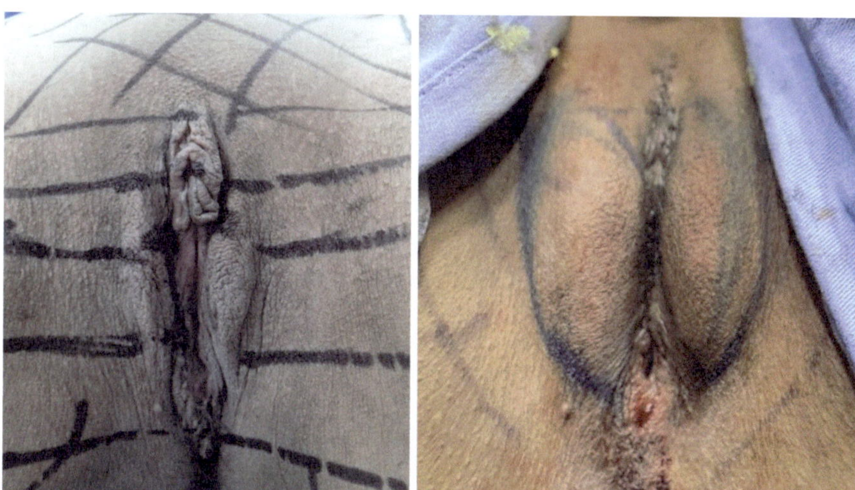

Fig. 7.2 Patient with significant loss of volume of the labia majora and a history of surgical amputation of the labia minora. Reconstruction of the labia minora is carried out, and in order to protect the vaginal entrance, 30 cc of macrofat is applied to each labia majora. (Photos courtesy of Dr. Pablo González Isaza)

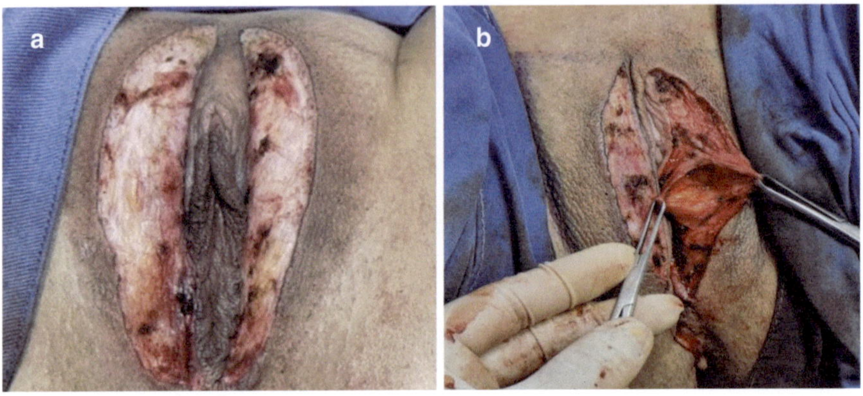

Fig. 7.3 (**a**) Skin resection of the labia majora with preservation of Dartos in the dissection. (**b**) Opening of the Dartos with excision of the fat pad to be resected to then reconstruct the Dartos wall and avoid herniation of deep tissues. (Photos courtesy of Dr. Pablo González Isaza)

7.2 Reduction of Fat Tissue of the Lavias Major

For very mild cases, liposuction of the labia majora can be considered using thin cannulas of up to 3 mm. In cases where the fat pad warrants it, it may be required to perform it in an open manner, incising the Dartos fascia, reducing the padding and also reconstructing the structures in planes to avoid herniations of the fat layer [1] (Fig. 7.3).

7.3 Dermolipectomy of Labia Majora

The most frequently used and accepted incision is on the medial edge of the labia majora lateral to the boundary between the labia majora and minora or interlabial fold. This wound allows hiding in the fold and also prevents hair translocation that can cause discomfort or dyspareunia.

Subsequently, a crescent is drawn that, using the pinch technique, can define how much tissue to remove in the anterior, middle, and posterior third and several according to the needs of each patient.

Additionally, as a recommendation, the wounds should not meet in the midline or at the commissure level or in the perineal body [1] (Fig. 7.4).

Reduction of the labia majora is indicated when the patient complains of excessive size and ptosis of the labia majora, becoming more visible when standing [11] (Fig. 7.5).

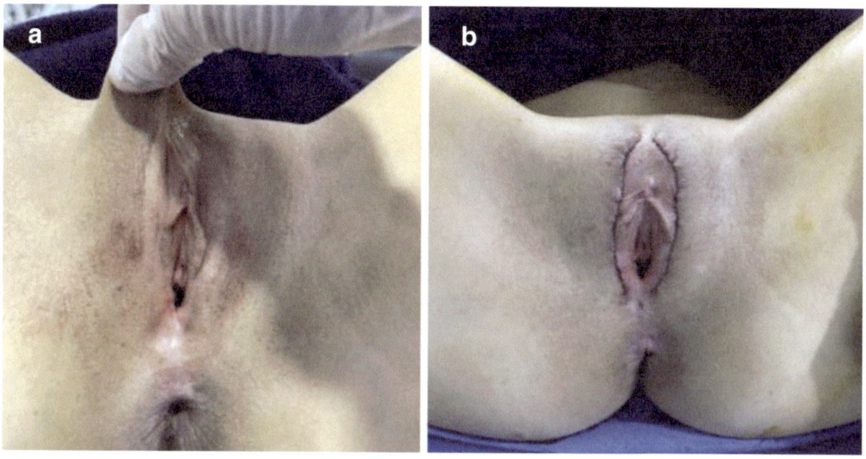

Fig. 7.4 (**a**) Pinch test to determine degree of laxity (**b**). Incisions in bilateral interlabial line after dermolipectomy

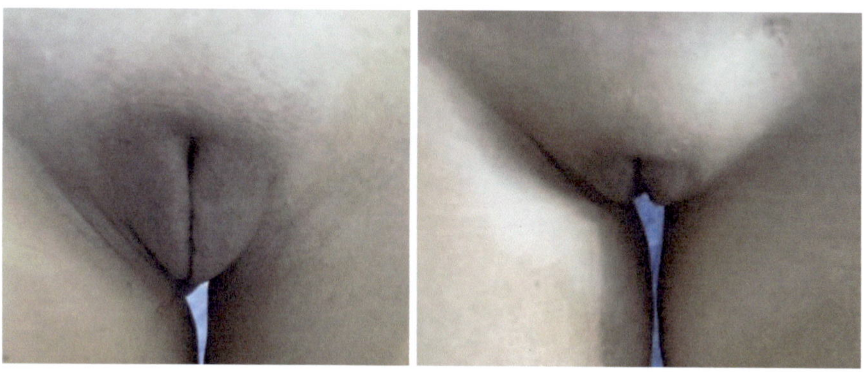

Fig. 7.5 Standing images of a patient with significant ptosis and hypermobility of the labia majora before and after the surgical procedure

7.4 Combined Treatments

If labiaplasty of the labia majora and minora is required at the same surgical time, the labia majora should be performed first since the anatomical characteristics of the labia minora change when the labia majora are intervened [12] (Fig. 7.6).

Other combined treatments may include Mons Venus interventions or liposuction with the procedures previously described [11] (Fig. 7.7).

Absolute contraindications

- Expectations that are not possible to meet with a surgical approach
- Blood dyscrasias

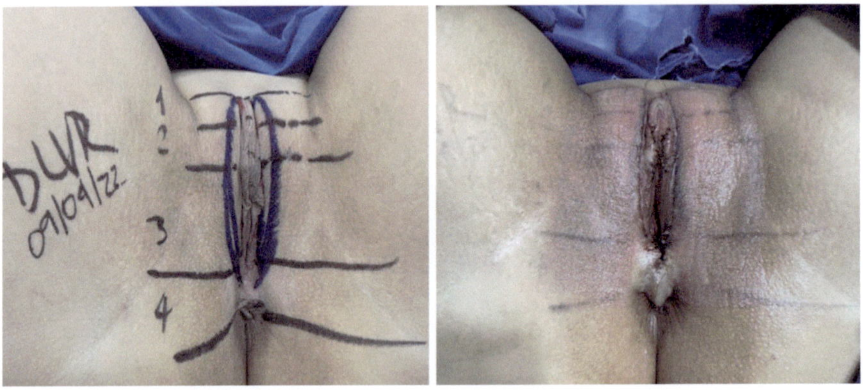

Fig. 7.6 Pre- and immediate postoperative images of combined labiaplasty of the labia majora and minora

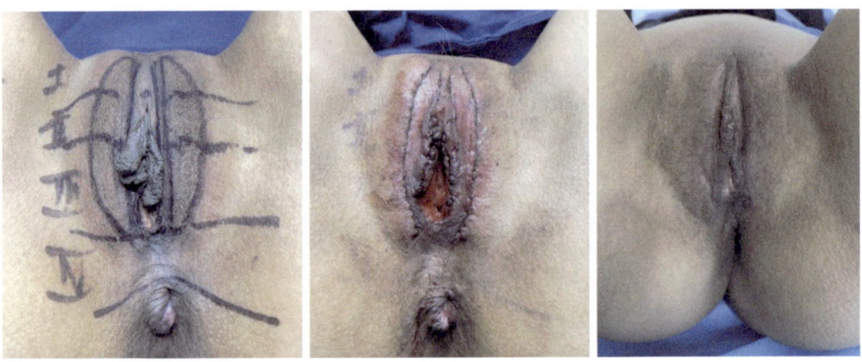

Fig. 7.7 Pre, immediate and 1-month postoperative images of combined labiaplasty of the labia majora and minora and Mons Venus lipoplasty

- Pregnancy and lactation
- Untreated varicose disease of the labia majora

Relative contraindications

- History of poor healing mainly in lateral incisions at the level of femoral folds
- Undiagnosed and untreated sexual dysfunction
- Smoking
- Untreated dysmorphism

Legal and ethical aspects

- Do not encourage surgery if the patient is not looking for it
- Be of legal age

- Keep in mind that by some organizations labiaplasty is considered an unnecessary procedure even if its purpose is to improve well-being and comply with the WHO definition of health.
- Completion and signing of informed consent including possible complications that may arise

When choosing surgical procedures on the labia majora, it is important to individualize each patient and be methodical in the choice of cases and procedures in order to have the best possible results.

References

1. Saheb-Al-Zamani M. Labia Majora reduction (Majoraplasty). Clin Plast Surg. 2022;49(4):489–94. https://doi.org/10.1016/j.cps.2022.06.010. PMID: 36162943.
2. Jabbour S, Kechichian E, Hersant B, Levan P, El Hachem L, Noel W, Nasr M. Labia Majora augmentation: a systematic review of the literature. Aesthet Surg J. 2017;37(10):1157–64. https://doi.org/10.1093/asj/sjx056. PMID: 28449124.
3. Salgado CJ, Tang JC, Desrosiers AE 3rd. Use of dermal fat graft for augmentation of the labia majora. J Plast Reconstr Aesthet Surg. 2012;65(2):267–70. https://doi.org/10.1016/j.bjps.2011.07.010. Epub 2011 Jul 30. PMID: 21803669.
4. Kotti B, Triana L, Condé-Green A, Janne Hasbun S, Cansancao AL, Agag RL. Assessment of female genital surgery education in plastic surgery training: report of an expert opinion survey. Aesth Plast Surg. 2019;43(4):1102–10. https://doi.org/10.1007/s00266-019-01394-6. Epub 2019 May 13.
5. Fasola E, Gazzola R. Labia Majora augmentation with hyaluronic acid filler: technique and results. Aesthet Surg J. 2016;36(10):1155–63. https://doi.org/10.1093/asj/sjw083. Epub 2016 May 30.
6. González-Isaza P, Wagner M, Hamori C, Rizo DV, Parra G, Guisantes E, Beltrán DM, Palacios S. Labia Majora approach to aesthetic and functional complaints. A standardized topographic labia Majora classification. Surg Technol Int. 2024;45:sti45/1834. Epub ahead of print. PMID: 39821916.
7. Seleem M, Osman OM, Kashmar SG, Lotfy R. Dimensions, ratios, volumes, and weights of the fatty parts of the vulva (Mons pubis and labia Majora). Aesthet Surg J. 2023;43(9):1002–12. https://doi.org/10.1093/asj/sjad106. PMID: 37067361.
8. Kang Y, Xia Z, Wang S, Yu N, Liu Z, Qin F, Zhang M, Wang X, Long X, Zhu L. Standardized photography of female genitalia and anatomical evaluations. Aesthet Surg J. 2023;43(11):1334–44. https://doi.org/10.1093/asj/sjad127.
9. Vogt PM, Herold C, Rennekampff HO. Autologous fat transplantation for labia majora reconstruction. Aesth Plast Surg. 2011;35(5):913–5. https://doi.org/10.1007/s00266-011-9664-5. Epub 2011 Feb 27.
10. Lapalorcia LM, Podda S, Campiglio G, Cordellini M. Labia majora labioplasty in HIV-related vaginal lipodystrophy: technique description and literature review. Aesth Plast Surg. 2013;37(4):711–4. https://doi.org/10.1007/s00266-013-0159-4. Epub 2013 Jun 15.
11. Alter GJ. Pubic contouring after massive weight loss in men and women: correction of hidden penis, Mons ptosis, and labia majora enlargement. Plast Reconstr Surg. 2012;130(4):936–47. https://doi.org/10.1097/PRS.0b013e318262f57d. PMID: 23018703.
12. Hersant B, Jabbour S, Noel W, Benadiba L, La Padula S, SidAhmed-Mezi M, Meningaud JP. Labia Majora augmentation combined with minimal labia Minora resection: a safe and global approach to the external female genitalia. Ann Plast Surg. 2018;80(4):323–7. https://doi.org/10.1097/SAP.0000000000001435. PMID: 29461295.

Chapter 8
Local Anesthesia Considerations for Labia Majoraplasty

Michael A. Reed and Red Alinsod

Key Points

- Selecting the right anesthesia technique is essential for both patient comfort and successful outcomes in office-based labia majoraplasty.
- Local anesthesia and tumescent anesthesia are safe, effective options for experienced practitioners in outpatient settings, offering patients a quicker recovery compared to general anesthesia.
- A pudendal block can provide targeted pain relief for the vulva and lower vagina, though careful technique is needed to avoid risks like vascular injection or incomplete anesthesia.
- Sedation, including anti-anxiety medications, can help calm patients, especially during initial injections, enhancing comfort throughout the procedure.
- Plasmaporation and dermoelectroporation are useful tools for increasing anesthetic absorption in labiaplasty and other vulvar procedures, allowing for deeper numbing and pigmentation reduction.
- Techniques for precise local infiltration, including using buffered solutions and avoiding high volumes, are important for minimizing discomfort, bleeding, and postoperative swelling.

M. A. Reed · R. Alinsod (✉)
Institute of Restorative and Cosmetic Gynecology, Davis, CA, USA

Alinsod Institute PLLC, Dallas, TX, USA
e-mail: red@gynflix.com

P. Gonzalez Isaza (ed.), *Aesthetic and Functional Alterations of the Labia Majora*, https://doi.org/10.1007/978-3-031-97405-2_8

8.1 Introduction

In office-based procedures like labia majoraplasty selecting the right anesthesia technique is key for both patient comfort and effective results. New surgeons may start by performing these procedures in hospitals with general anesthesia. However, experienced practitioners can safely perform vulvar procedures in an outpatient clinic using local or tumescent anesthesia, offering patients a less invasive option with faster recovery times.

There are various anesthesia options: general anesthesia, spinal blocks, regional blocks, or local anesthesia, sometimes with mild sedation. Each technique has benefits and specific applications, such as pudendal blocks for localized pain relief in the vulva and lower vagina. Numbing solutions can be customized to each patient, and techniques like plasmaporation and dermoelectroporation can improve anesthetic absorption for procedures like labiaplasty and vaginoplasty. This chapter outlines these approaches, offering a safe, effective anesthesia framework tailored for labia majoraplasty.

8.2 Regional Block

A pudendal block is a useful and effective way to numb the vulva and lower vagina, making it a good option for labia majoraplasty. However, it is not necessary in most cases and spotty in results. This type of anesthesia can be ideal for patients comfortable with it and for doctors experienced in the technique. I typically use about 5–10 mL of 0.25–0.5% bupivacaine with epinephrine and bicarbonate on each side, providing pain relief that lasts 3–5 hours. However, there are some challenges with pudendal blocks, including the risk of hitting a blood vessel, injuring a nerve, or not fully numbing the area.

Sedation can help reduce anxiety, especially at the start of a procedure when the patient is awake. An antianxiety medication or a mild pain reliever might also be appropriate. Before performing a labia majoraplasty in an office setting, I typically give the patient 1 mg of lorazepam by mouth 30–45 minutes before surgery once all questions are answered and consents signed. If needed, another 1 mg can be given under the tongue shortly before prep, depending on the patient's comfort and input from the nurse. Oral narcotics such as 25–50 mg of meperidine (Demerol) or 2 mg of hydromorphone (Dilaudid) 30 minutes before cut time can also help relax and give the patient a warm fuzzy feeling that the patients find comforting. The addition of 4 mg of ondansetron (Zofran) or 10 mg of prochlorperazine (Compazine) can help reduce nausea also and aid in the gentle sedation without Intravenous sedation (IVs).

Other types of antianxiety meds or pain relievers, and different doses, can be used depending on the patient's needs. Furthermore, patients are also instructed to drink fluids and eat a light meal before arriving to prevent low blood pressure after the procedure. Since they are awake and alert, they can continue to sip water to stay hydrated during the case.

8.3 Local Infiltrative Process

The local infiltrative process begins with 10–20 minutes of electroporation (aka **plasmaporation, predictive permeation, and dermoelectroporation)** using a 30% Benzocaine-Lidocaine-Tetracaine (BLT) numbing cream**.** Electroporation is a technique that can be used both on the outer labial skin and inside the vaginal canal. It is helpful for lightening skin tones, reducing pigmentation, and enhancing the effect of topical anesthetics before procedures like labia majoraplasty, vaginoplasty, and other vagina/vulvar procedures. Only 1–5 milliamperes of energy is used making it exceptionally safe.

Researchers found that applying a quick electric field to a cell makes its outer membrane temporarily open, allowing larger molecules to pass through. In this case we are pushing the 30% numbing cream deep under the skin. This technique, called electroporation, lowers the skin's resistance and opens water channels, enabling deeper absorption of therapeutic agents. Within 30 minutes, the pores naturally close, safely trapping the treatment in the target cells without harming them. Electroporation is now used in labia majoraplasty to deliver active numbing ingredients effectively through the vulvar skin (1). A recent innovation using DC current called Plasmaporation has also been shown to be very effective (Figs. 8.1, 8.2, 8.3, 8.4, 8.5, and 8.6).

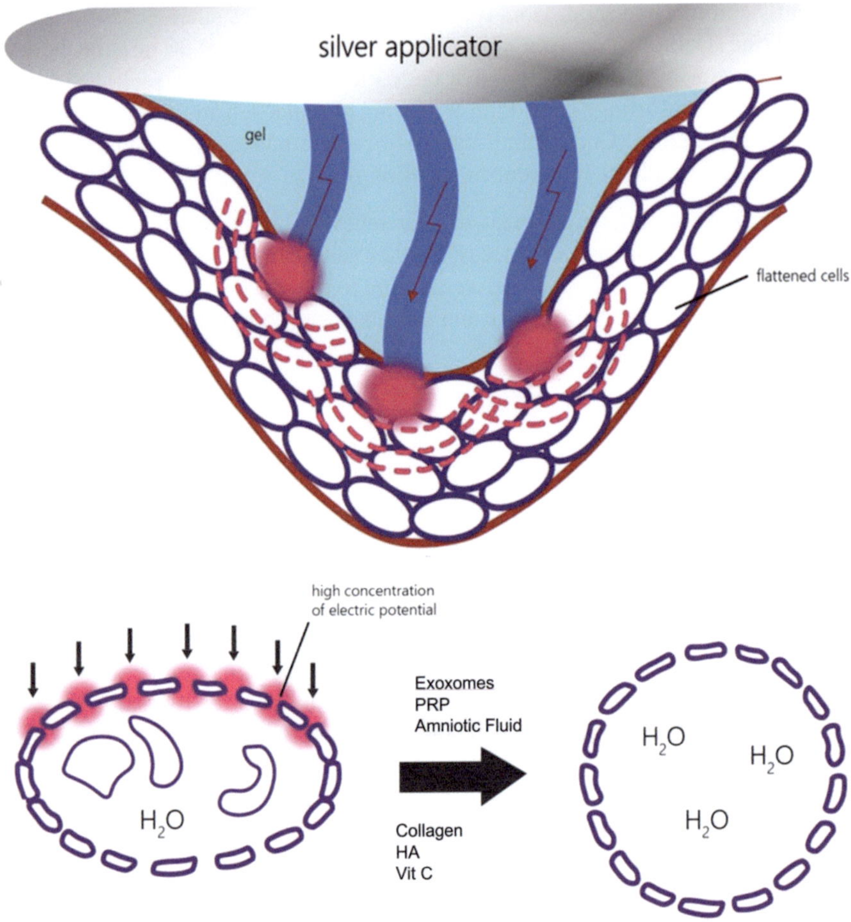

Fig. 8.1 Opening of the skin's water channels with milliampere DC allows the placement of topical anesthesia deep under the skin without the use of needles

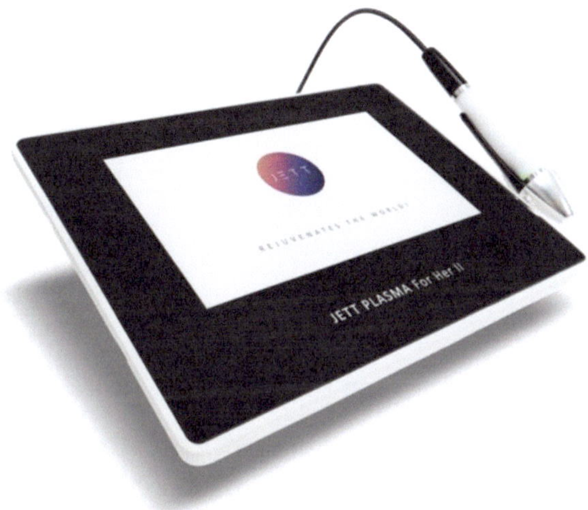

Fig. 8.2 Compex Jett plasma

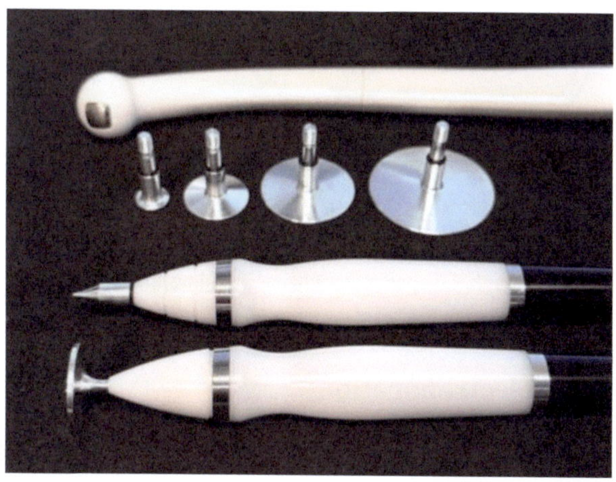

Fig. 8.3 Tips and wands

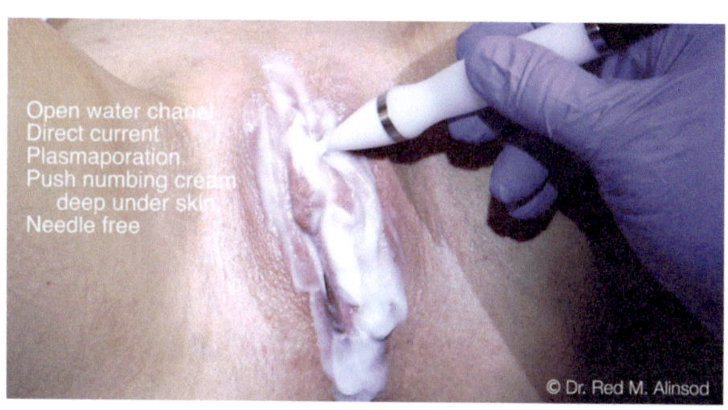

Fig. 8.4 Ten minutes of topical treatment into the surgical sites

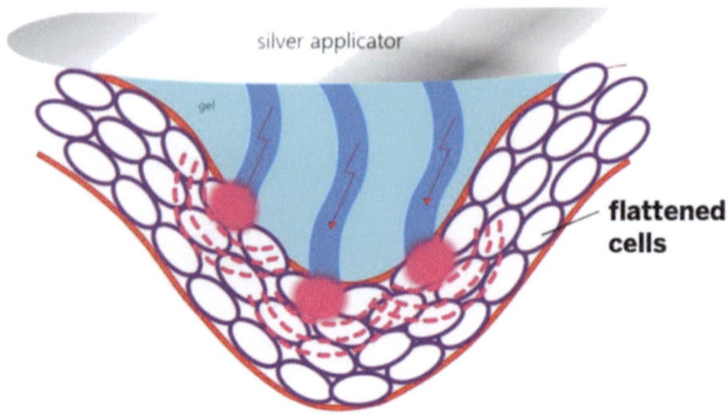

Fig. 8.5 Plasma energy is created right over the skin and opens the water channels

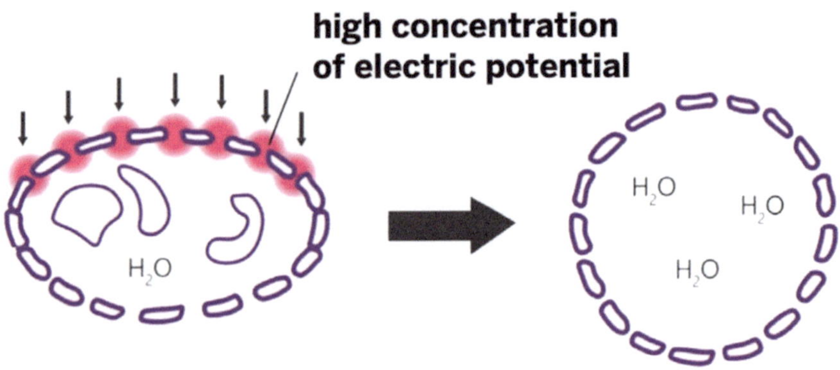

Fig. 8.6 Molecules such as water, topical anesthesia, PRP, exosomes, vitamin C, and collagen, are pushed through the open water channels and trapped inside the cell

8.4 Electroporation

8.4.1 Plasmaporation

My general approach is to begin the local infiltrative process by first using electroporation prior to local injection for numbing during office-based labia majoraplasty. This method is reliable and very safe and provides long-lasting numbing. Any local anesthetic can be used, with or without epinephrine, depending on the patient's needs. My preference is 0.25% bupivacaine with epinephrine (Fig. 7). It is important to avoid injecting directly into blood vessels and not to exceed safe dosages: 30 mL of 0.5% bupivacaine or 60 mL of 0.25%. All local anesthetics are injected retrograde in manner.

Local anesthetics are acidic, so they can sting. This can be reduced by adding a small amount of sodium bicarbonate to the solution (Fig. 8.7). Using too much

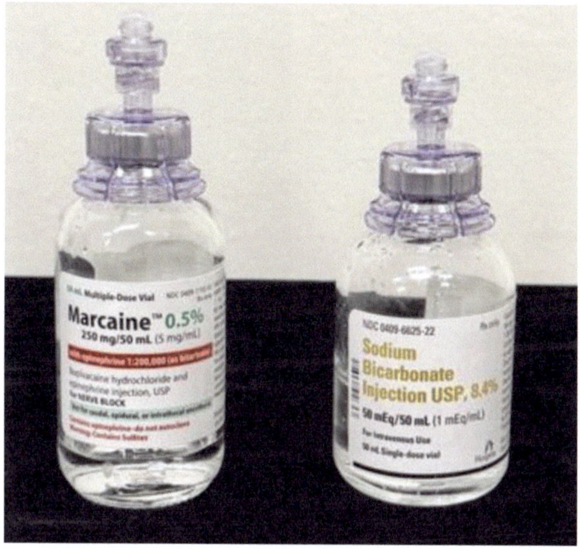

Fig. 8.7 Bupivacaine and bicarbonate

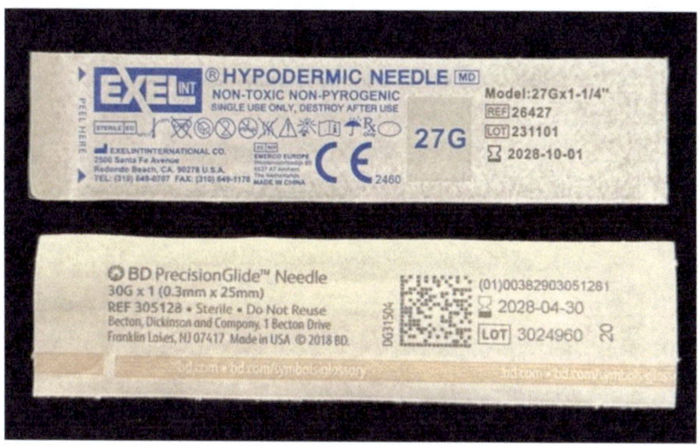

Fig. 8.8 27-gauge 1.25″ needle and 30-gauge 1″ needle

anesthetic can make it harder to control bleeding during surgery. The more anesthetic used, especially when combined with electrocautery, the higher the risk of tissue damage, which can lead to excessive swelling, discomfort, and changes to the skin. This can impact the overall results of the procedure. Dr. Alinsod uses 6 cc of 0.5% bupivacaine with 4 cc of bicarbonate for a total of 10 cc of a cloudy solution. This mix dramatically reduces the burning sensation. You will need many 30 gauge needles because the bicarbonate crystal can clog the tips. A 1-inch 30-gauge or 1.25-inch 27-gauge needle will work well (Fig. 8.8).

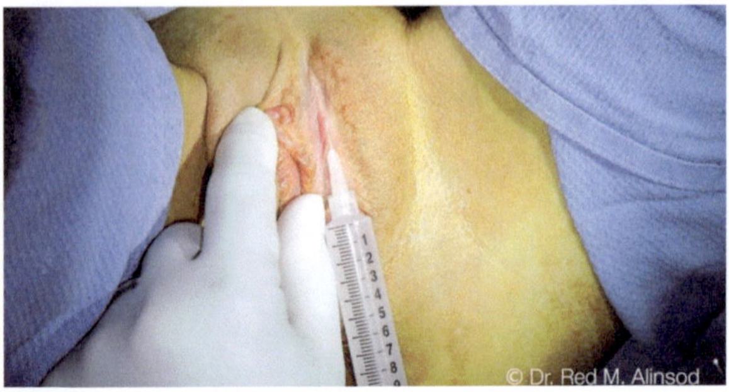

Fig. 8.9 Local anesthesia on the crease and ridges of the labia majora

8.5 Labia Majoraplasty Numbing Technique

To prepare for majoraplasty, a mixture of local anesthetic and sodium bicarbonate is drawn into a 10-mL syringe with a 27- or 30-gauge needle. Local infiltration begins at the top level of the clitoral hood and continues into the interlabial fold which lies between the lateral labia majora and the medial clitoral hood and labia minora. The infiltration is carried down the entire interlabial fold to the level of the introitus (Fig. 8.9). Next local is injected by starting again at the top of the interlabial fold and extending laterally just past the top ridge of the labia majora, curving back down toward the lowest point of the introits. This is repeated on the contralateral side.

While the patient is awake, supportive measures like nitrous oxide or "handholding" by a nurse or assistant can help ease anxiety. Patients are informed beforehand about the short-lasting discomfort during injection, which typically lasts less than 30–60 seconds per side. The injection may be done in short 20-second intervals, counted out to the patient by the surgeon or assistant. Before starting the incision, the area is checked with forceps or needle tip to ensure complete numbing, allowing about 5 min for the anesthetic to fully take effect.

On average, 8–10 mL of anesthetic is used (up to 10 cc per side), depending on the surgical area's complexity and if a clitoral hood reduction is included. You will need double to triple that for fat pad removal. Unless you are very experienced in office-based anesthesia, I recommend fat pad removals to be done in a surgery center under general anesthesia with the use of Exparel at the end of the case.

At the very end of the case, you can also inject 20 cc of liposome coated bupivacaine (Exparel) for pain control averaging 3 days. It is expensive but well worth it for the traveling patient. The 20 cc of Exparel is typically mixed 50:50 with injectable saline for a total of 40 cc volume of fluid. Warning: Exparel burns when injected, so warn the patient. Exparel burns when injected and does not act as rapidly as standard bupivacaine, so I do not use it at the start of the case. The liposome coat is deactivated by lidocaine, so do not use lidocaine at all when using Exparel. You can add bicarbonate to Exparel, but I have seen less efficacy when this is done.

In summary, choosing the right anesthesia method for office-based labia majoraplasty significantly impacts both patient comfort and procedural success. With experience, local and tumescent anesthesia options become powerful tools for creating a safe and relaxed environment outside the hospital setting. Techniques like pudendal blocks, sedation, electroporation, and local infiltration each offer distinct advantages for specific needs, allowing tailored approaches to anesthesia that maximize comfort and efficiency. This chapter highlights these diverse anesthesia options, providing a comprehensive framework for practitioners to deliver effective, patient-centered care in aesthetic vulvar procedures.

8.6 Disclosure

The authors of this chapter have no commercial or financial conflicts.

Reference

1. Hamori C, Banwell PE, Alinsod RM. Female cosmetic genital surgery. Thieme; 2017.

Chapter 9
Surgical Instrumentation for Labia Majora Labiaplasty

Ana Maria Gutierrez

More and more functional and psychosocial disorders are presented due to a hypo- or hypertrophy of the labia majora, causing multiple disorders such as discomfort to perform any exercise or even walking, hygienic difficulties, pain, and discomfort with underwear and in some cases discomfort carrying a pleasant sexual intercourse.

The appearance of labia majora not only varies from woman to woman but also influences the age, race, the number of births, and hormonal conditions of each one; this can be solved with a surgical intervention named labia majora labiaplasty which reduces excess of skin and in some increases their size with the purpose to improve the appearance obtaining a more rejuvenated and aesthetic appearance.

With this surgery, different benefits are achieved that cover not only the aesthetic but also the functional part, being the proposal to improve the quality of life of patients.

Next, the supplies and instruments used to perform such surgery will be mentioned.

9.1 Materials

Applicators
Hypodermic needles # 18, 25 or 27, and 30 mm
Methylene blue
Scalpel blade #15
Stockinette
Gauze and compresses
Gloves

A. M. Gutierrez (✉)
Private Operating Room Calculaser, Pereira, Colombia

P. Gonzalez Isaza (ed.), *Aesthetic and Functional Alterations of the Labia Majora*, https://doi.org/10.1007/978-3-031-97405-2_9

3, 5, 10, and 20 cm syringes
Micropore
Electro pencil and pediatric electro tip
Clothing package
Ruler
Saline solution
Infiltration medications: plain bupivacaine, lidocaine without epinephrine, and tranexamic acid
Centrifuge for platelet-rich plasma (PRP) to be processed at the center

9.2 Sutures

1. Vicryl rapide (polyglactin 910): This suture is a synthetic, sterile, absorbable suture composed of a copolymer consisting of 90% glycolide and 10% L-lactide.

   Colorless, braided
   Used in 5/0-gauge 45 cm length with P-1 3/8 needle, 11 mm cutter 3/8.
   Strength retention profile: 50% in 5 days and 0% in 14 days
   Absorption time: 42 days

2. Chromic catgut: It is an absorbable chromic catgut suture, monofilament, beige color.

   It is composed of purified connective tissue, especially collagen, derived from the serosal layer of bovine or the submucosal fibrous layer of sheep intestines.
   Strength retention profile: 21–28 days
   Absorption time: 90 days

3. Silk: Braided suture, multifilament, of protein nature, obtained from silkworm cocoon fibers, it is black in color for easy visibility and impregnated with beeswax, and it has high flexibility and tensile strength.

9.3 Surgical Instruments

A surgical instrument is defined as a tool or implement designed to perform specific actions during surgery, but this concept encompasses much more.

We need to focus on what kind of instruments we require to meet the needs of each procedure.

For this purpose, they have been classified into four main groups:

Hemostasis instruments: They are used to grasp and hold tissues or blood vessels.
Apprehension instruments: These are used to grasp the tissues or blood vessels.

Dieresis instruments: These are the instruments used to make the incision or section of the tissues.
Suture instruments: These are the instruments that join the tissues allowing their continuity.

In addition, we must consider other characteristics such as the material with which they are manufactured since some can be made of titanium, or other metals, although the vast majority, are made of surgical steel, so their care must comply with all maintenance standards and must undergo the process of cleaning and disinfection.

They should also be a great tool to help the surgeon to perform all surgical maneuvers during surgery.

It is the responsibility of all those who handle the surgical instruments to ensure that they are maintained and used properly and that their average useful life is increased.

For the surgical technique of labiaplasty we will have a table which we will dress with a sterile field, and on it we will place all the necessary supplies, sutures, and instruments.

9.4 Hemostasis Instruments

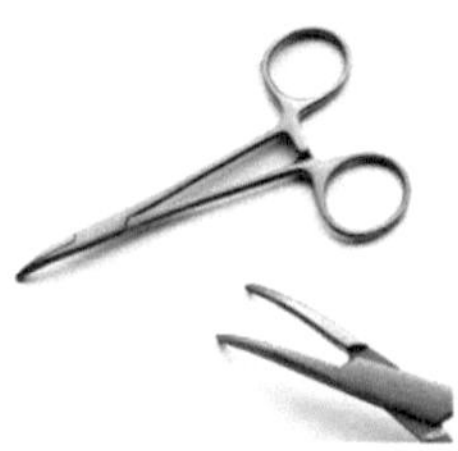

Curved mini clamp

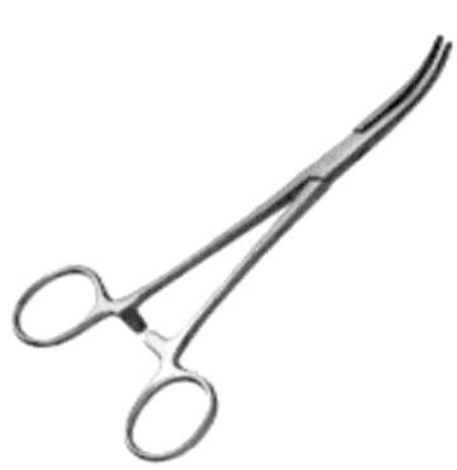

Curved Kelly clamp

9.5 Holding Instruments

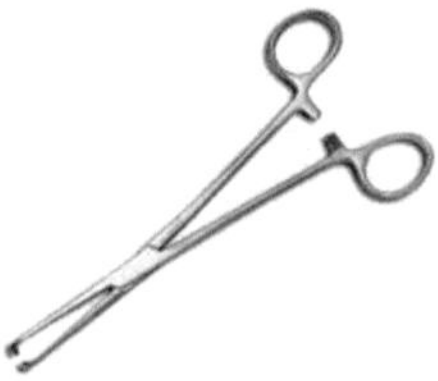

Allis clamp

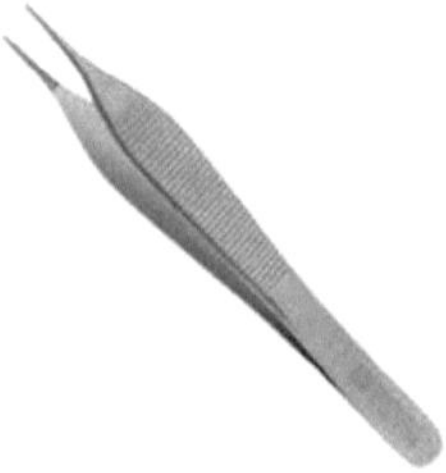

Adson clamp

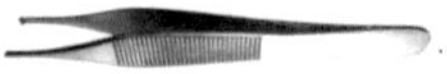

Toothed Adson clamp

9.6 Cutting Instruments

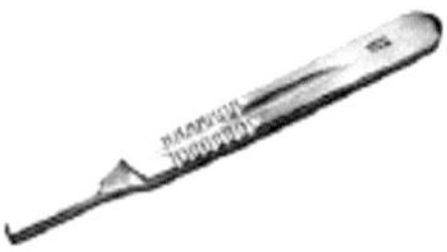

Scalpel holder # 3

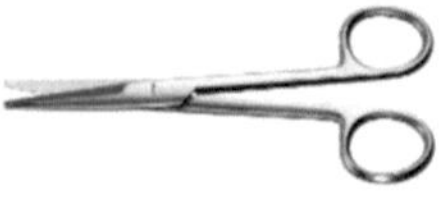

Mayo scissor

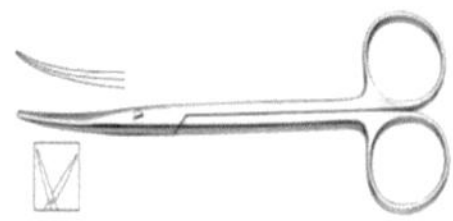

Curved Metzenbaum scissor

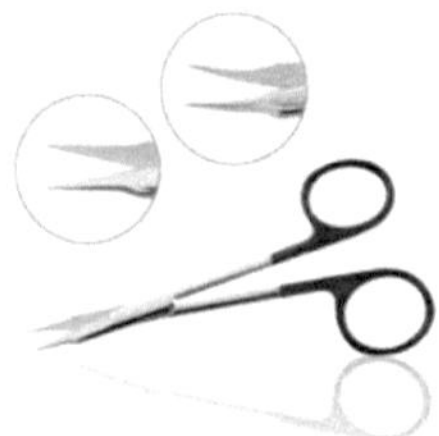

Stevens scissor

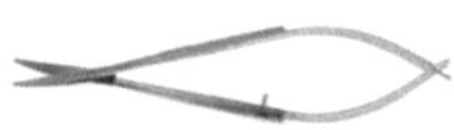

Castroviejo scissor

9.7 Suturing Instruments

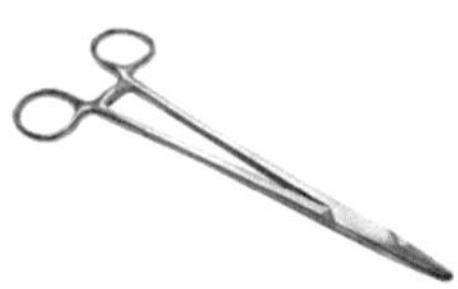

Mayo-Hegar needle holder

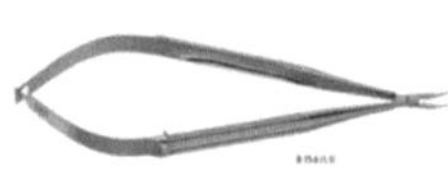

Castroviejo needle holder

9.8 Basic ACCESORIES

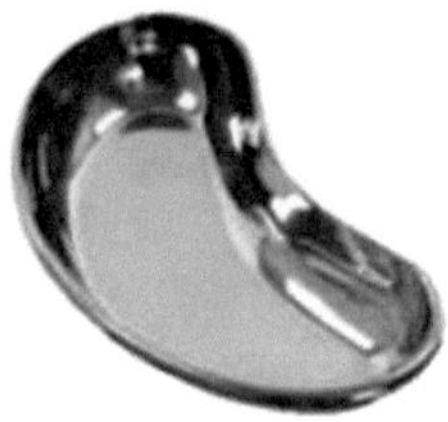

Container

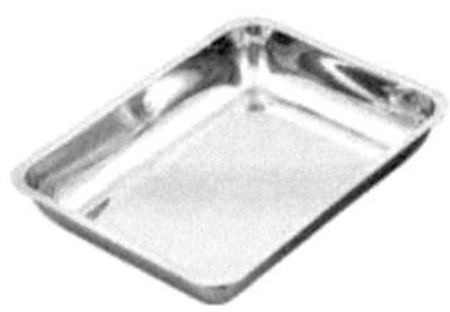

Tray

Chapter 10
Role of Energy Based Devices (EBD) Energy Sources, for Labia Majora Aesthetic and Functional Concerns

Pablo Gonzalez Isaza

One of the most popular and effective alternatives for the approach of labia majora aesthetic and functional alterations is the use of energy-based devices. Skin laxity is a challenging situation that necessarily demands the use of sources that deliver energy in different ways, to heat to deep structures such as the endopelvic fascia which contributes to tightening of labia majora.

Deep heating delivered energy into the labia majora stimulates collagen production through a controlled wound healing response that occurs over time; this collagen remodelling yields the desired tissue tightening that is seen with selected energy-based devices [1].

Radiofrequency-based energy devices offer great results regarding labia majora laxity improvement with a non-invasive approach, and this energy is a form of electromagnetic current that can be delivered through special probes to labia majora, and when applied to the underlying skin and soft tissue, it generates contraction by the rupture of hydrogen bonds in the collagen structure generating shortening and thickening of the collagen fibrils; afterwards a wound healing cascade stimulates neo angiogenesis, collagenesis, and elastin formation in the following months [2].

Inside our centre our first experience was with the use of monopolar RF (Thermiva).

Figures 10.1 and 10.2. This device is based on monopolar emission of radiofrequency through a special probe designed to treat vagina and vulvar area, the treatment times are usually around 10 min per each labia majora, and it can be performed by paramedic personnel due to the simplicity of application and safety, which is related to thermistors inside the probe that give the applier information in real time about the actual temperature applied to the tissue avoiding burns and discomfort.

P. Gonzalez Isaza (✉)
Obstetrics and Gynecology, Urogynecology Minimally Invasive Surgery,
Hospital Universitario San Jorge, Pereira, Colombia

Soranus Center for Funtional and Regenerative Urogynecology, Pereira, Colombia

P. Gonzalez Isaza (ed.), *Aesthetic and Functional Alterations of the Labia Majora*, https://doi.org/10.1007/978-3-031-97405-2_10

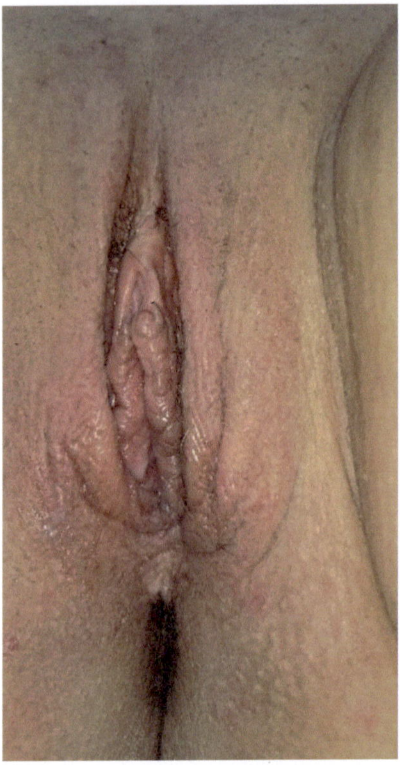

Fig. 10.1 Before TTCRF

After around three sessions with 2- to 3-week interval, patients report improvement of skin laxity and high degree of satisfaction.

We consider important to differentiate the technological aspects of probes from this devices, specifically regarding the polarity, there are plenty of options inside the market regarding probe design, polarity, and number of electrodes, and in simple terms there are only three possibilities: monopolar, bipolar, and multipolar which is indeed a bipolar configuration but with added electrodes to improve adherence to the tissue, ergonomics, and simply a marketing strategy from companies (Fig. 10.3).

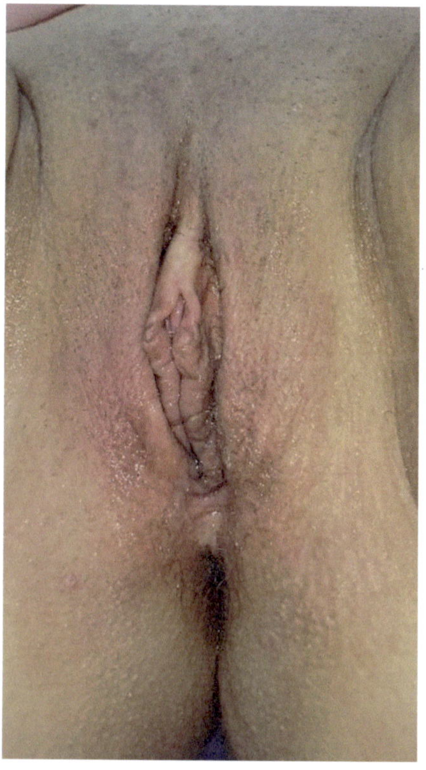

Fig. 10.2 After first session of TTCRF

Monopolar RF has a contact electrode with the tissue and another electrode that is usually very far away from it, usually a plaque that is in contact with hips or feet. This way is usually what is considered in electro-coagulator because it is permitting a higher flux of current, necessary for vaporizing the tissue. In this methodology it is very difficult to foresee where the current is passing through and potentially more dangerous; in contrast bipolar RF is emitted between two electrodes that are usually very close (maximum distance few millimetres). The electrical current is passing from one electrode to the other, and there are no possibilities to go around the body; in this way we are absolutely sure that current is confined just between the electrodes [3].

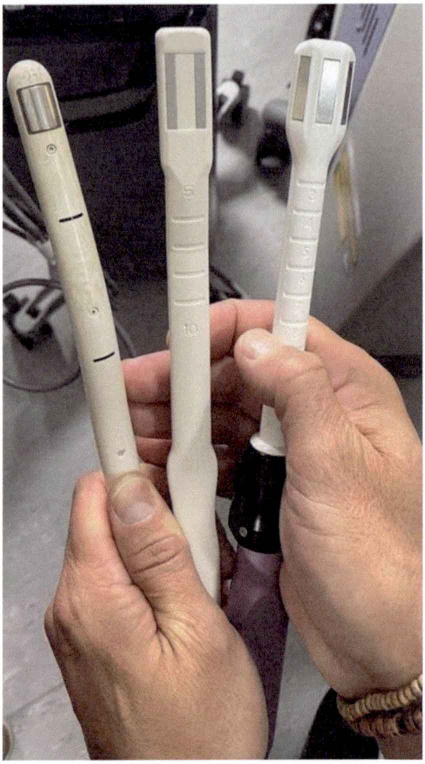

Fig. 10.3 Probes with different polarity, from right to left: monopolar, bipolar, and multipolar

10.1 Importance of the Technique

According to our anatomical findings in the cadaver dissections, labia majora laxity is related not only to skin alterations but also to deeper structures such as the fascia, traditionally practitioners when performing radiofrequency-based treatments in labia majora, only focus on the labial corpus, which is wrong, and there are other fascial components such as Colles, campers, and Scarpa, which in healthy conditions offer different vectors of traction called (puboclitoral, crural, gluteal, and perineal expansions) (Fig. 10.4).

That is why inside our protocol we extend the movement of the probe to all these areas, so more tissue can be stimulated by the heat emission.

We have noticed improvement of skin laxity according to the pinch test after the bipolar RF protocol (Fig. 10.6), this strategy is very easy, safe, and effective, and it can even be applied by paramedic personnel (Fig. 10.5).

Inside our centre we always use validated questionnaires and scales to objectively evaluate vulvar skin laxity before and after any energy-based device treatment, the vulvar skin assessment scale is a validated and useful tool for these conditions, and we used it inside a short follow-up of ten patients treated with bipolar radiofrequency (Fig. 10.6).

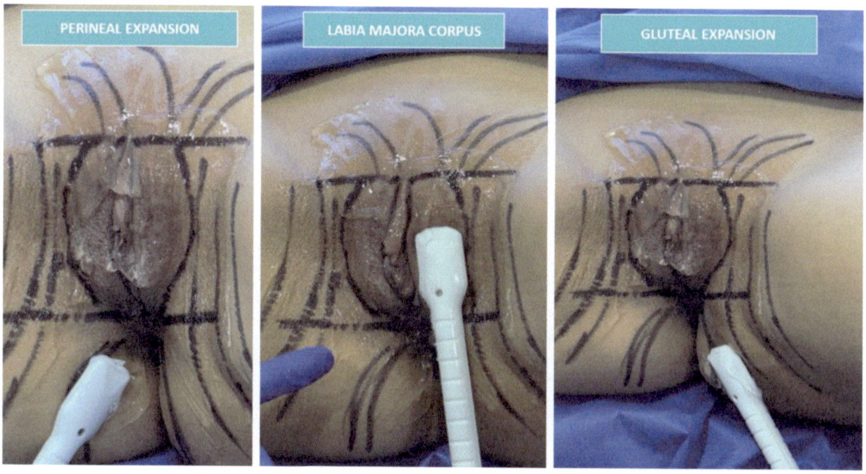

Fig. 10.4 Expansions of fascia perineal, labial corpus, and gluteal for suggested probe movement

Fig. 10.5 Bipolar radiofrequency for labia majora skin laxity applied by paramedic personnel

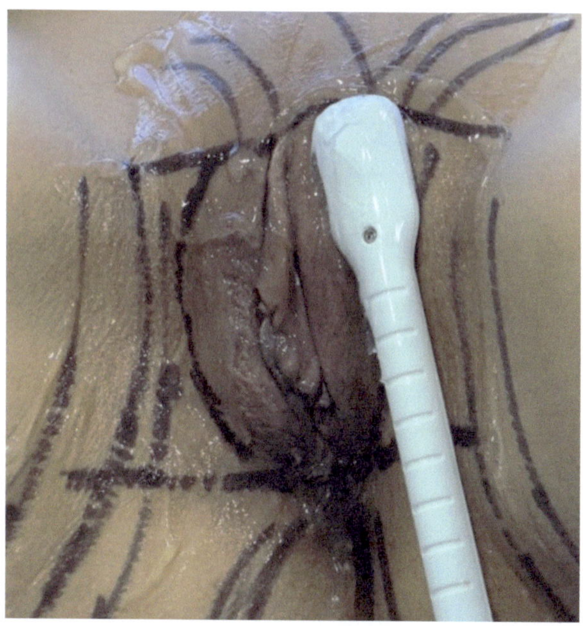

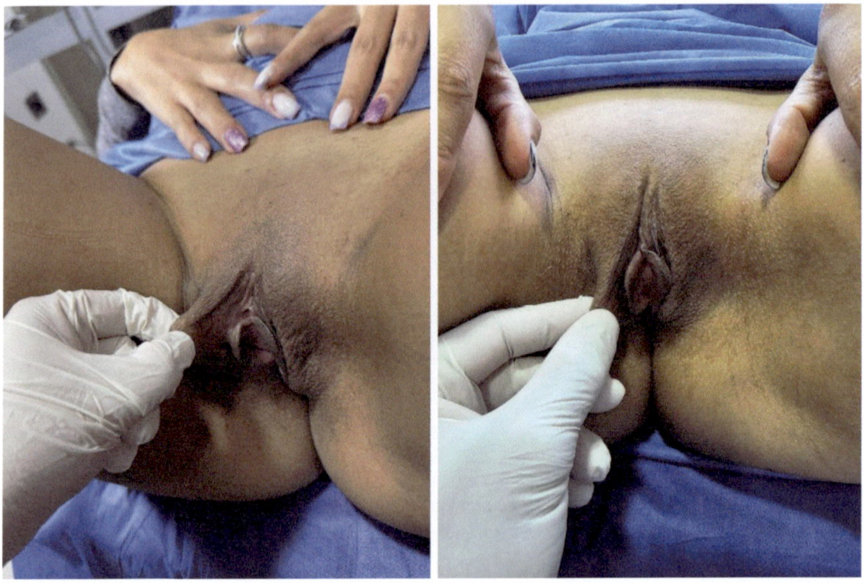

Fig. 10.6 Improvement of skin laxity according to the pinch test after the bipolar RF protocol

The improvement of scores from baseline to the end of the treatment (and Forma-V Inmode) was noticeable (Fig. 10.7).

Another important option for labia majora aesthetic and functional conditions is related to the use of fractional needle delivered radiofrequency, and there are quite a lot of options inside this market; anyhow technology, safety, and effectiveness play a big role regarding patient results. Our most important experience regarding this type of technology is with the use of a specialized device that has the ability to deliver energy in a very precise way, meaning that laxity, atrophy, or lipodystrophy conditions can be approached by just modifying settings regarding depth and fractional energy delivery inside this platform, in selected cases besides laxity there is also a need to improve skin quality, and we use calcium hydroxyapatite 0.001% as a collagen stimulator added to the radiofrequency treatment (Fig. 10.8a-b).

For more severe cases of skin laxity, there are other options, which have been traditionally used by plastic surgeons and aesthetic medicine practitioners, such as the endolift procedure, and it can be performed with either Nd-Yag (1064 nm) laser or diode (980–1470 nm) laser; these devices demand a large learning curve and offer potential complications such as burns, because they are operator-dependant, and the procedure can be performed either in office with tumescent solution or inside the operator room under general anaesthesia. A 300–600 nm optical fibre guided by a microcannula is inserted parallel to the anterior vulvar commissure at the apex of both labia majora, and according to the anatomy,1500–2000 joules are delivered inside dartos fascia, to generate tissue contraction and after some weeks a noticeable skin tightening effect.

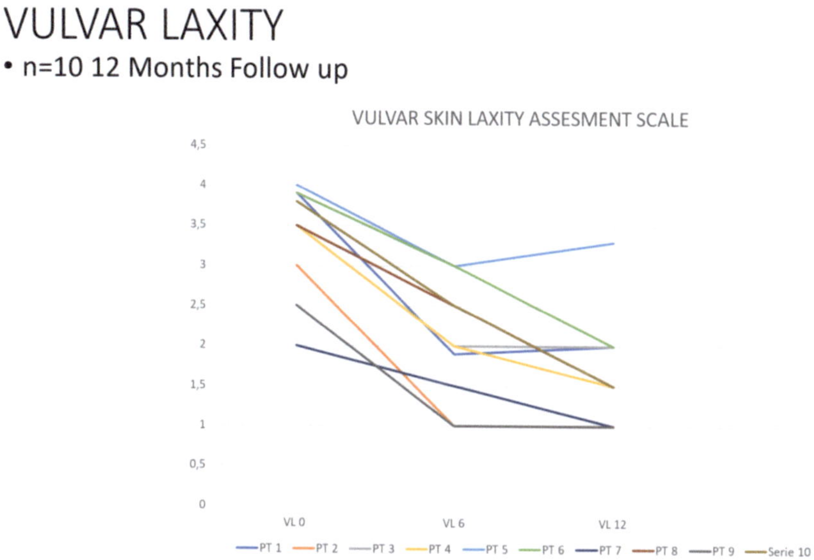

Fig. 10.7 Vulvar skin laxity assessment scale before and after bipolar radiofrequency (Forma-v Inmode)

In the past years we used an Nd-Yag laser (1064 nm) to treat lipodystrophy and laxity conditions in labia majora, and the results were acceptable, but touch-up sessions were needed to achieve desired results (Fig. 10.9a–b).

A more recent approach to improve more severe cases of labia majora hyperlaxity is related to the use of minimally invasive techniques such as bipolar temperature-controlled radiofrequency also named dielectric radiofrequency that heat tissues around 36 °C externally and 63 °C internally (Fig. 10.10a–b). This heat emission leads to neocollagenesis, angiogenesis, and elastogenesis over the next months leading to a marked improvement of skin laxity in labia majora [5].

According to a recent review of non-invasive devices for skin tightening, clinicians must have a good patient selection to have better results; also same authors believe that radiofrequency technology is superior to laser regarding aesthetic results, in a safer way [4].

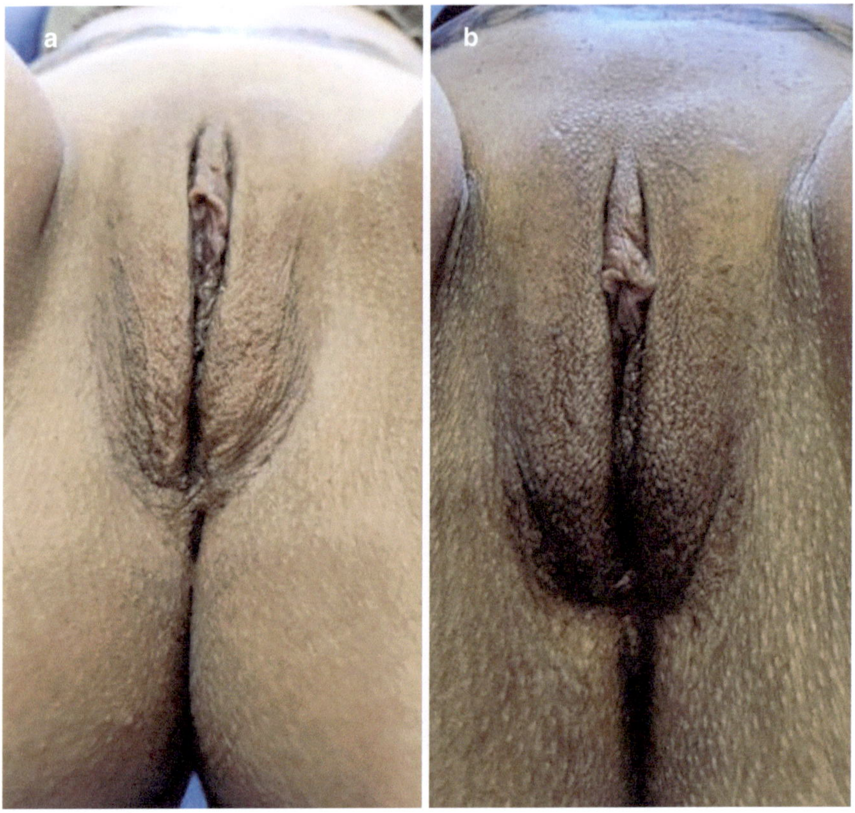

Fig. 10.8 (**a, b**) Before and after fractional needle radiofrequency (Morpheus-8)in combination with calcium hydroxyapatite 0.001% as a collagen stimulator for skin improvement

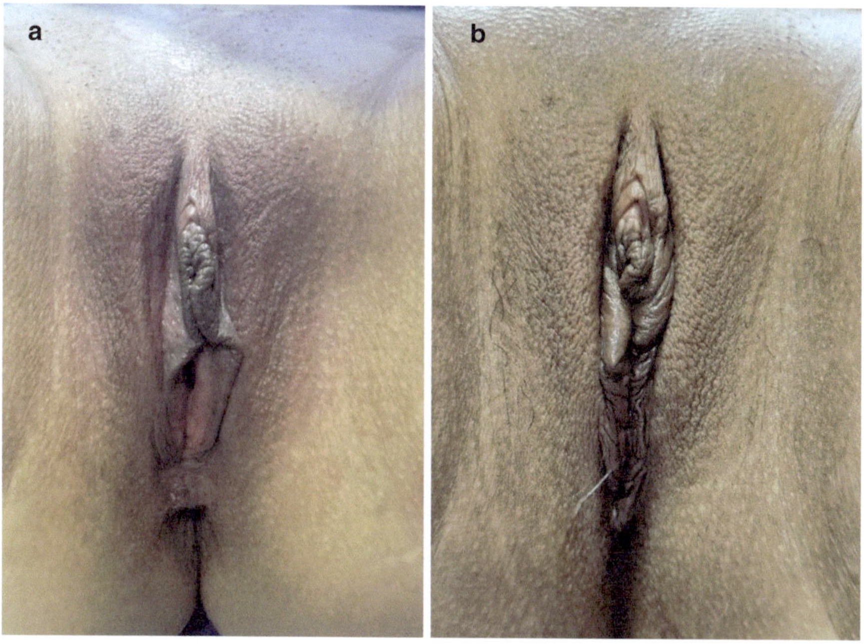

Fig. 10.9 (**a–b**) Labia majora endolifting with Nd-Yag laser (1064 nm) before and after 6 weeks

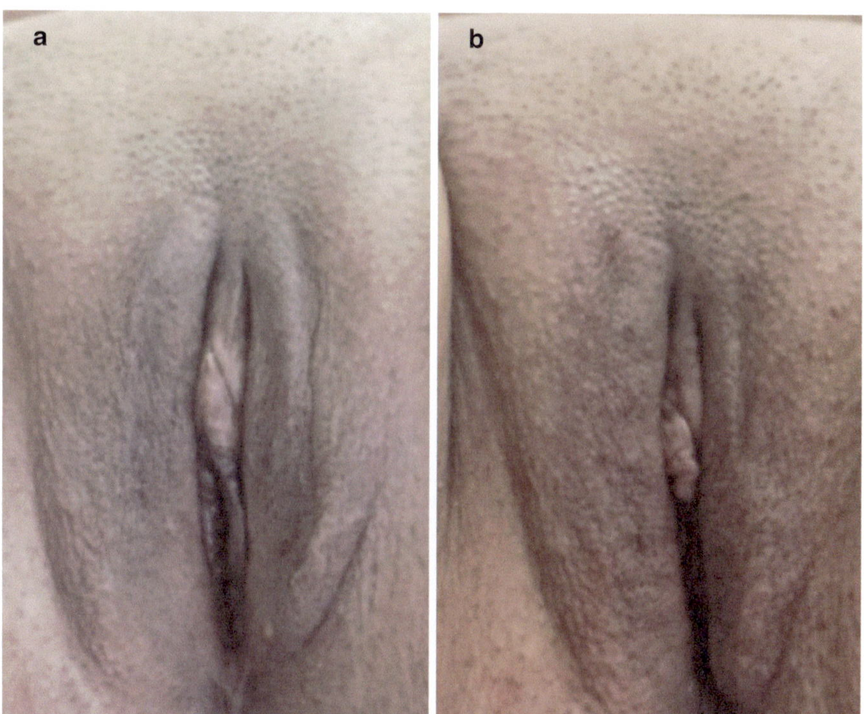

Fig. 10.10 (**a–b**) Labia majora endolifting dielectric radiofrequency 1.5 k/joules per side on labia majora before and after 60 days

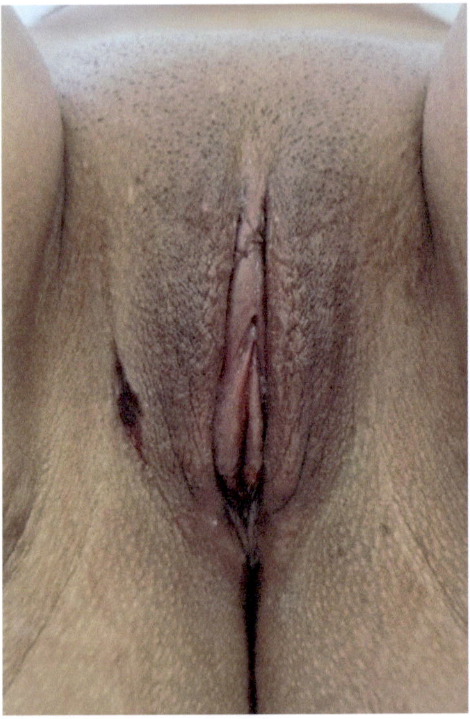

Fig. 10.11 Bipolar radiofrequency burn in a patient under general anaesthesia

10.2 Complications

The most common complication is related to burns, due to deficient technique, unproper technology, or rarely when the procedure is performed under sedation or general anaesthesia this last scenario, and basically there is no patient feedback regarding the temperature tolerance (Fig. 10.11).

References

1. Dierickx CC. The role of deep heating for noninvasive skin rejuvenation. Lasers Surg Med. 2006;38:799–807.
2. Zelickson BD, Kist D, Bernstein E, et al. Histological and ultrastructural evaluation of the effects of a radiofrequency-based nonablative dermal remodeling device: a pilot study. Arch Dermatol. 2004;140:204–9.
3. Isaza PG, Rizo DV, Garibay I, Galvan R. The role of bipolar radiofrequency (Bprf) as a mechanism of bio-stimulation for the treatment of Vulvo-vaginal laxity: a novel approach. Int J Clin Exp Med Res. 2021;5(3):367–76.

4. Mazzoni D, Lin MJ, Dubin DP, Khorasani H. Review of non-invasive body contouring devices for fat reduction, skin tightening and muscle definition. Australas J Dermatol. 2019;60(4):278–83. https://doi.org/10.1111/ajd.13090. Epub 2019 Jun 6. PMID: 31168833.
5. Dayan E, Ramirez H, Theodorou S. Radiofrequency treatment of labia Minora and Majora: a minimally invasive approach to vulva restoration. Plast Reconstr Surg Glob Open. 2020;8(4):e2418. https://doi.org/10.1097/GOX.0000000000002418. PMID: 32440388; PMCID: PMC7209841

Chapter 11
Complications in Labia Majoraplasty: A Guide to Prevention and Treatment

Michael A. Reed and Red Alinsod

Key Points

- Proper patient selection for excision versus filling or both.
- Office versus surgery center depends on anxiety levels.
- Meticulous surgical technique is critical to preventing complications such as hematoma formation, wound breakdown, and scalloping of surgical edges.
- Pain, bruising, and edema can be effectively managed through a combination of icing, medications, and adjunct therapies to accelerate healing.
- Proper suture selection and placement reduce the risks of premature absorption, wound dehiscence, and excessive scarring.
- Patient adherence to postoperative guidelines plays a major role in preventing wound breakdown and ensuring optimal healing.
- Recognizing and managing nerve-related discomfort through preoperative counseling and targeted treatments like local estrogen application can improve patient experience.
- Early recognition and prompt treatment of infections and complications are essential to preventing escalation, ensuring a smooth recovery, and enhancing overall patient satisfaction.

M. A. Reed · R. Alinsod (✉)
Institute of Restorative and Cosmetic Gynecology, Davis, CA, USA

Alinsod Institute PLLC, Dallas, TX, USA
e-mail: red@gynflix.com

P. Gonzalez Isaza (ed.), *Aesthetic and Functional Alterations of the Labia Majora*, https://doi.org/10.1007/978-3-031-97405-2_11

11.1 Introduction

Labia majoraplasty is a surgical procedure aimed at improving the aesthetic and functional aspects of the labia majora. While advancements in surgical techniques have led to increased patient satisfaction and improved outcomes, complications remain a possibility. Successful postoperative recovery depends on multiple factors, including precise surgical execution, thorough patient education, and vigilant postoperative care. Recognizing potential complications early and implementing effective prevention and management strategies are essential to minimizing risks and optimizing surgical outcomes.

This chapter explores the most common complications associated with labia majoraplasty, including pain, bruising, edema, hematoma formation, wound dehiscence, hypersensitivity, and scarring. Additionally, it provides evidence-based approaches for preventing and addressing these issues. A comprehensive understanding of these complications allows surgeons to refine their techniques, counsel patients effectively, and ultimately enhance both functional and aesthetic results.

11.2 Patient Selection

Careful patient selection is essential in determining whether excision, filling, or a combination of both is appropriate. Patients with loose, sagging labia majora are typically ideal candidates for surgical excision, whereas those experiencing volume loss without significant excess skin may benefit more from labial augmentation using fat grafting or platelet-rich plasma (PRP) combined with hyaluronic acid (HA). Figs. 11.1 and 11.2 show both laxity and deflation of the labia majora.

Over-resection in patients with minimal labial fat can result in an overly flat appearance, which may be desirable for some—such as athletes and highly active individuals—but not for others. Aesthetic preferences often vary by cultural background, with European and Middle Eastern women frequently favoring a fuller, more contoured labial appearance, while many women in California and other fitness-focused regions prefer a sleeker, more athletic look. These considerations should be thoroughly discussed during preoperative consultations to align surgical planning with the patient's desired outcome. In some cases, combining a conservative excision with mild vulvar augmentation may provide the most balanced and natural-looking result. Managing patient expectations and thoroughly explaining the pros and cons of excision versus augmentation ensure informed decision-making and satisfaction with the final outcome.

Fig. 11.1 Laxity

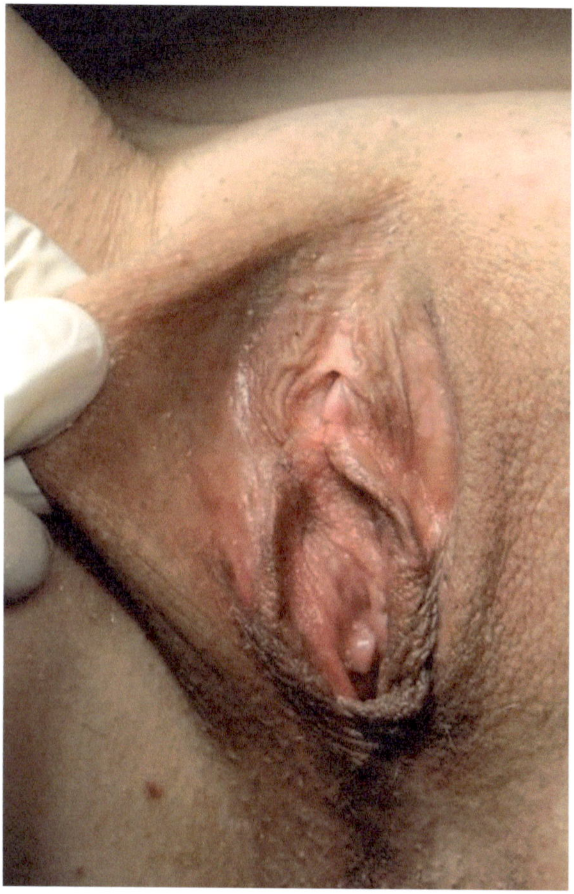

A secondary issue to consider is if a standard labia majoraplasty will suffice for patients with a great deal of fat pad beneath the skin. Removal of only the skin, as in a standard vulvectomy, will leave the patient with tighter skin but still with a prominent majora. Those patients may benefit more with a labia majoraplasty with fat pad removal as shown in Figs. 11.3, 11.4, 11.5, 11.6, and 11.7, resulting in a more petite and less prominent labia majora.

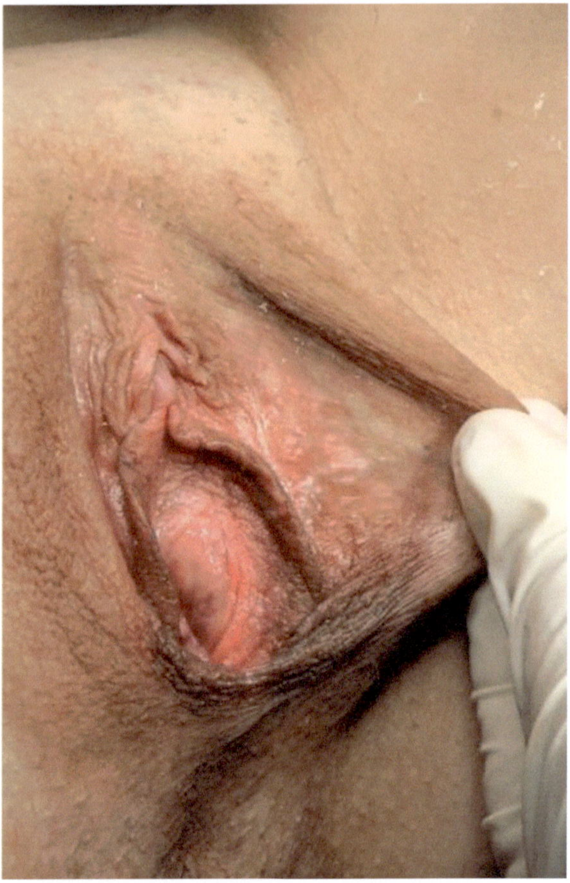

Fig. 11.2 Deflation

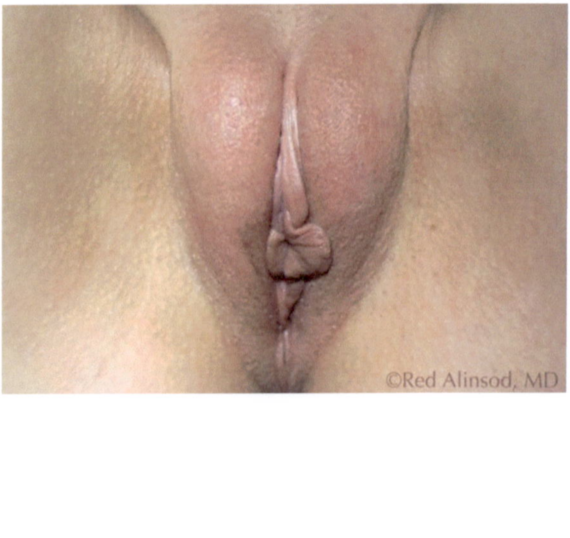

Fig. 11.3 Excess fat pad

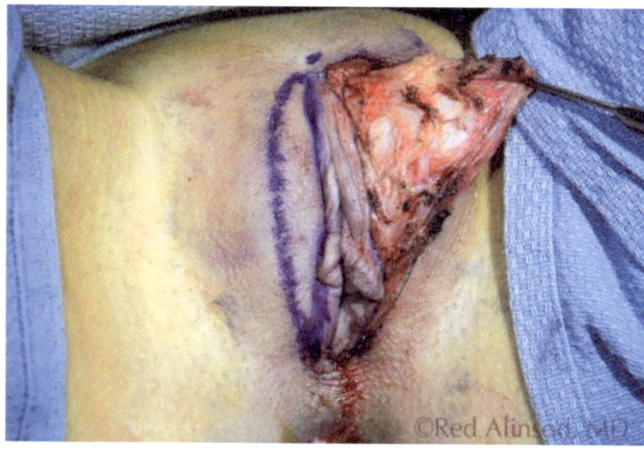

Fig. 11.4 Fat pad excision

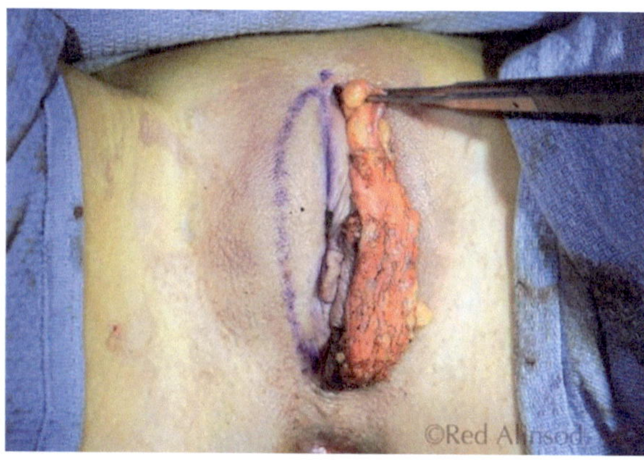

Fig. 11.5 Fat pad excised

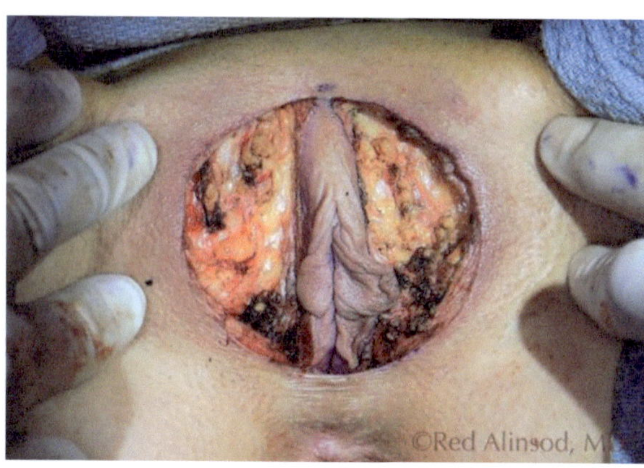

Fig. 11.6 Excess fat removed

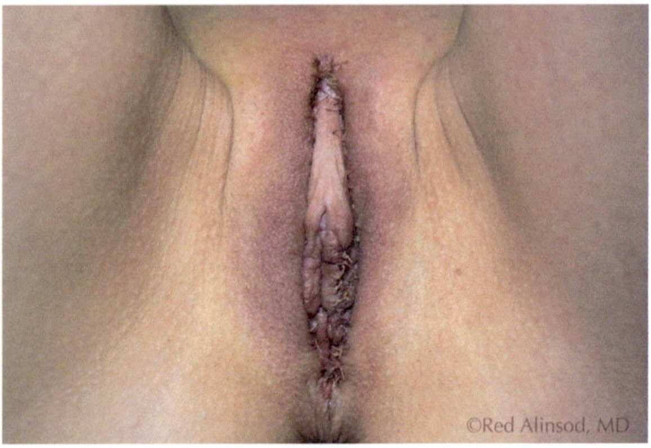

Fig. 11.7 Less majora prominence and a more athletic appearance

11.3 Location of Surgery and Management of Anxiety

The surgical setting plays a crucial role in patient comfort and anxiety management. The decision to perform labia majoraplasty in an office-based procedure room versus a surgery center should be guided by the patient's level of anxiety and overall tolerance for in-office procedures. Patients with a significant history of anxiety, panic attacks, or difficulty tolerating minor procedures may be better suited for surgery under general or regional anesthesia in a controlled surgical facility. Conducting the procedure in an office setting requires careful patient selection to ensure they can remain comfortable under local anesthesia with mild sedation.

For patients undergoing in-office procedures, preoperative anxiolytics combined with mild analgesics and anti-nausea medications can help ease discomfort and maintain relaxation. A commonly used regimen includes oral lorazepam in combination with meperidine or hydromorphone, supplemented with ondansetron to prevent nausea. This approach ensures that patients remain calm throughout the procedure while avoiding the risks associated with general anesthesia. Surgeons should carefully assess each patient's ability to tolerate an awake procedure and adjust their approach accordingly to minimize intraoperative anxiety and discomfort.

11.4 Pain, Bruising, and Edema

Postoperative pain, bruising, and edema are common but manageable aspects of recovery, as seen in Fig. 11.8. To minimize discomfort and swelling, patients should apply covered ice to the surgical site as frequently as possible during waking hours

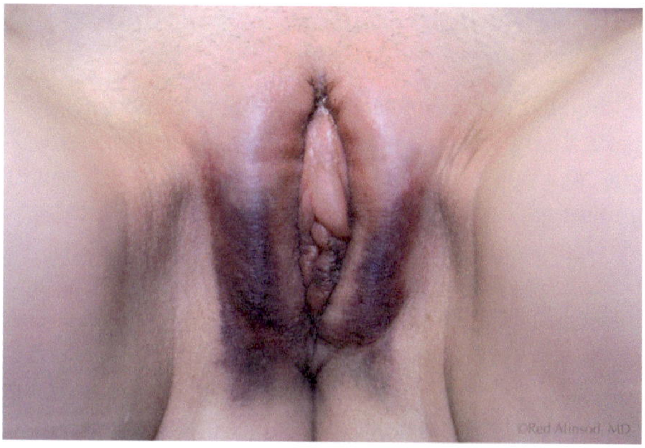

Fig. 11.8 Postoperative pain, bruising, and edema are common but manageable aspects of recovery

for the first seven days, with a minimum of four to five sessions per day. There should be no direct ice contact. Pharmacologic management includes prescribing pain medications such as tramadol or hydrocodone, in combination with an NSAID like ibuprofen, naproxen, and ketorolac. Patients should adhere to a strict medication regimen for at least the first 36 hours, after which they can transition to as-needed use.

Adjunct therapies can further aid in recovery. Arnica gel or cream, a homeopathic anti-inflammatory, helps reduce bruising and swelling, while Cu-3 cream promotes tissue hydration and repair. For surface discomfort, dermoplast spray or diphenhydramine cream can provide relief from itching and stinging when applied to external incisions. BLT (bupivacaine/lidocaine/tetracaine) compounded cream, between 20 and 30%, can also ease discomfort. Additionally, carboxy therapy gel (CO2LiftV by Lumisque) serves as a topical "hyperbaric oxygen chamber," stimulating collagen, elastin, and new blood vessel formation while reducing edema and ecchymosis, effectively shortening the healing process by up to 10 days [1].

11.5 Bleeding and Hematoma Formation

Preventing bleeding complications begins intraoperatively with meticulous hemostasis, conservative use of cautery, and layered suturing to eliminate dead space. Despite these precautions, hematomas can occasionally develop and must be addressed promptly. They will typically occur in the lower third of the labia majora, as shown in Fig. 11.8. Left untreated, a hematoma can serve as a nidus for infection, potentially leading to urethral obstruction or progressive expansion [2]. In such cases, surgical evacuation is recommended to mitigate these risks and promote proper wound healing.

11.6 Premature Suture Absorption and Wound Breakdown

Although rare, premature suture absorption occurs in approximately 4–7% of cases, particularly when braided sutures such as Vicryl are used. Closing in a single subcuticular layer significantly increases the risk of wound dehiscence. To prevent this, a multilayered closure is essential. Monofilament sutures such as Monocryl should be incorporated into the deeper tissue layers, offering longer-lasting structural support. Wound dehiscence commonly results from inadequate closure techniques or premature physical activity that places undue stress on the healing tissues. A proper closure should include a deep approximation layer to eliminate dead space, followed by a secondary layer to reinforce the wound edges without excessive tension. Clear pre- and postoperative instructions emphasizing restricted movement and adherence to a tension-free recovery period of 4–6 weeks are critical in preventing this complication. Patients should be advised to maintain their knees close together as much as possible to minimize tension across the incision site, facilitating proper wound healing. This "Velcro Knees" approach, as described by Dr. Alinsod, is particularly useful in reducing stress on healing tissues and applies to both labia majoraplasty and perineal repairs.

Here is an example of wound breakdown, granuloma formation, repair, and postoperative appearance in Figs. 11.9, 11.10, 11.11, 11.12, 11.13, 11.14, 11.15, and 11.16.

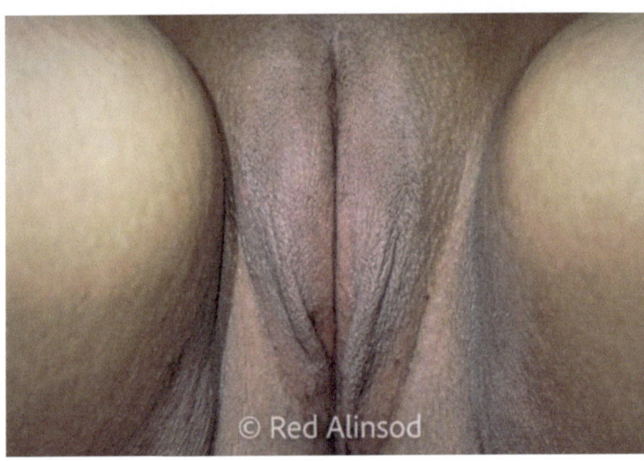

Fig. 11.9 Before surgery

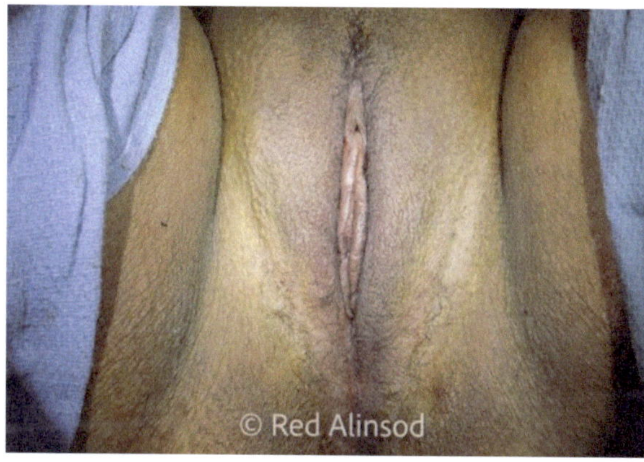

Fig. 11.10 Immediately after surgery

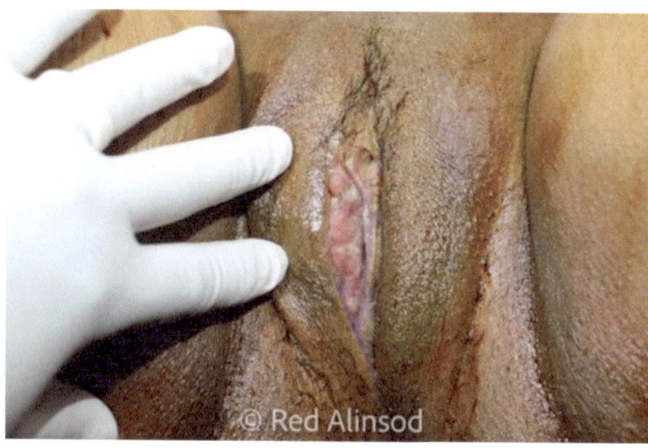

Fig. 11.11 Granuloma formation

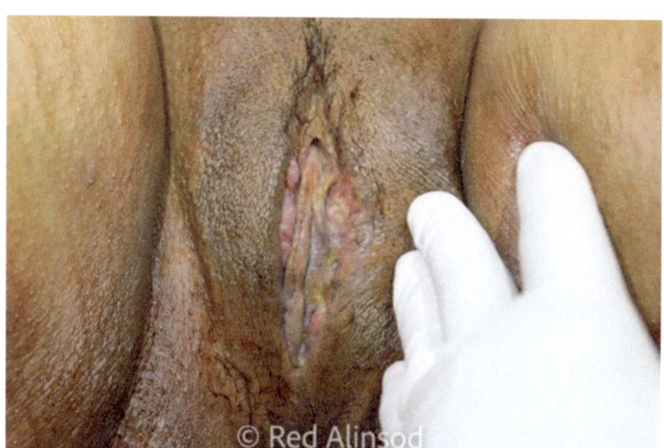

Fig. 11.12 Wound breakdown

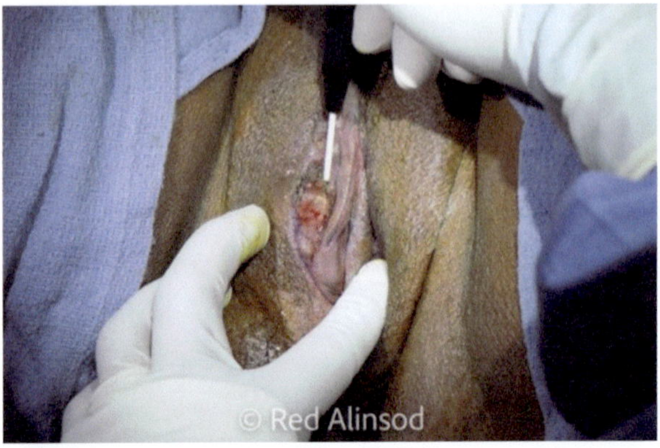

Fig. 11.13 RF excision of granuloma

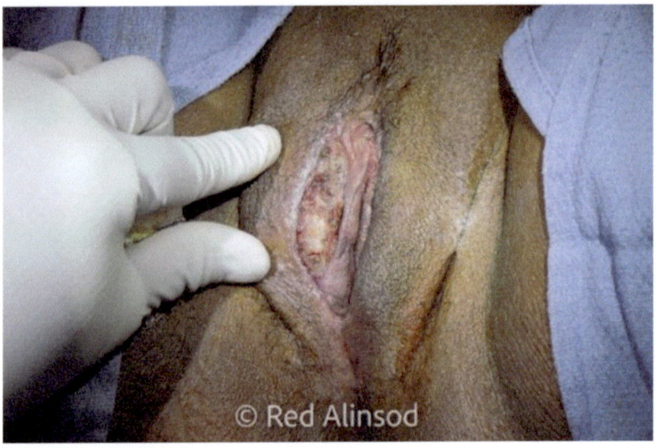

Fig. 11.14 Granuloma excised

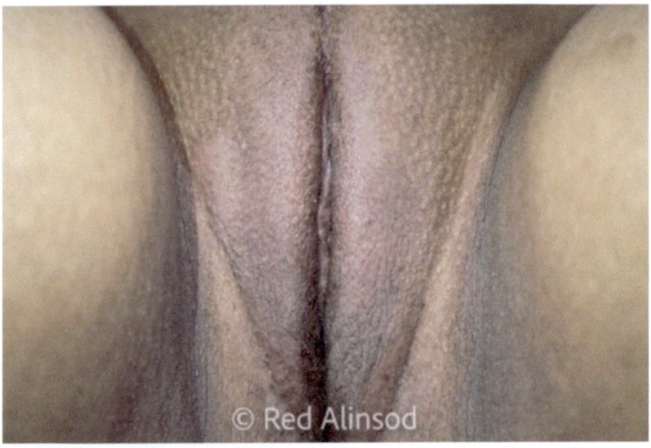

Fig. 11.15 Edges resutured

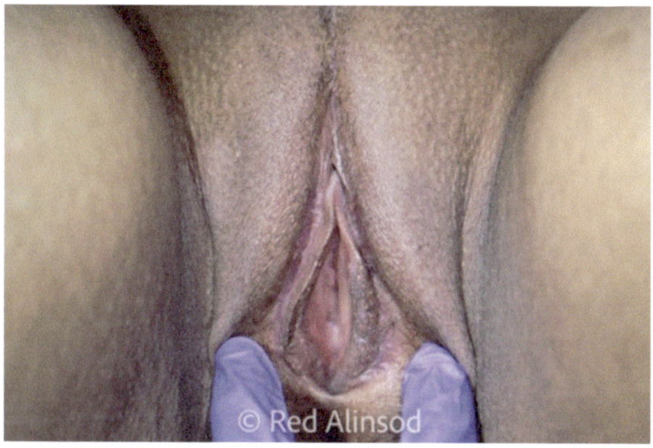

Fig. 11.16 Healed wound edges

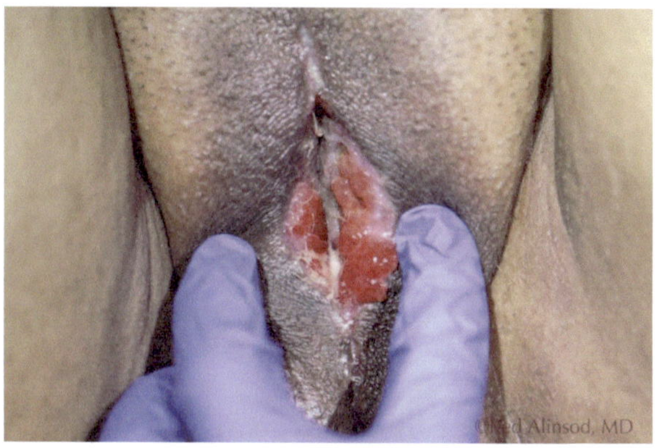

Fig. 11.17 Wound granuloma from wound breakdown

11.7 Wound Granuloma

Rare wound granulomas may occur when one-layer closures are performed that break down and expose the raw edges of the wound site. The use of estrogen cream on this area may eliminate these raised and red areas over time. If they form a raised polypoid structure, they may have to be surgically excised and oversewn like this example below in Figs. 11.17 and 11.18.

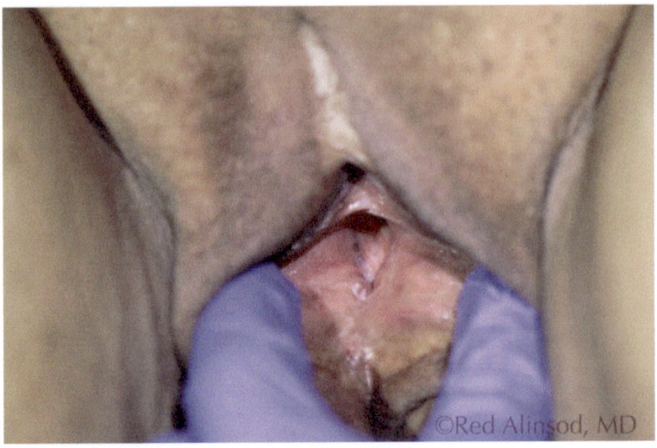

Fig. 11.18 Wound healed after excision of granuloma with resuturing

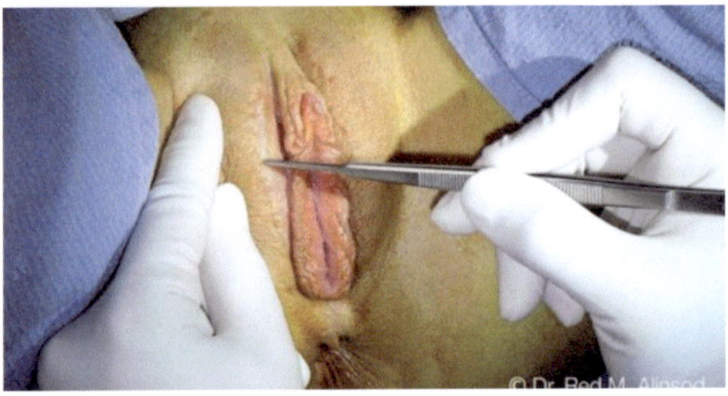

Fig. 11.19 Scar prominent

11.8 Visible Site of Surgical Scar

A visible scar may occur of the incision lines are not tucked in right next to the labia minora. This can be avoided by ensuring the suture lines are right at the base of the labia minora. The patient below had a prior labia majoraplasty where the incision line was not placed directly adjacent to the labia minora. The suture line is prominent at the top ridge of the labia majora in the example below: Figs. 11.19 and 11.20. In Fig. 11.21 the suture lines are placed more medial and adjunct to the labia minora and are invisible in the crease.

In this example below the prominent scars have been excised and tucked medially right next to the labia minora.

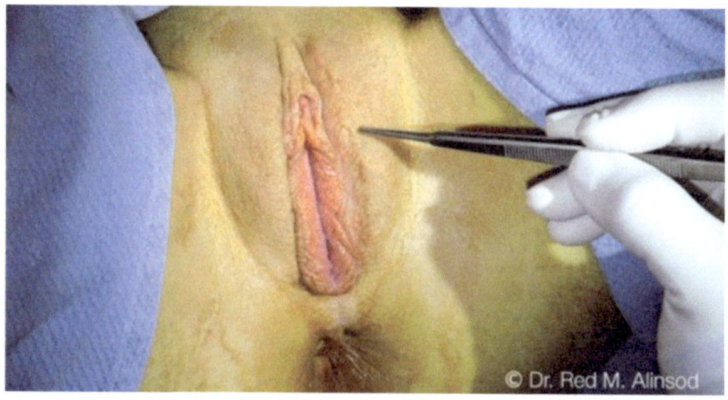

Fig. 11.20 Scar prominent

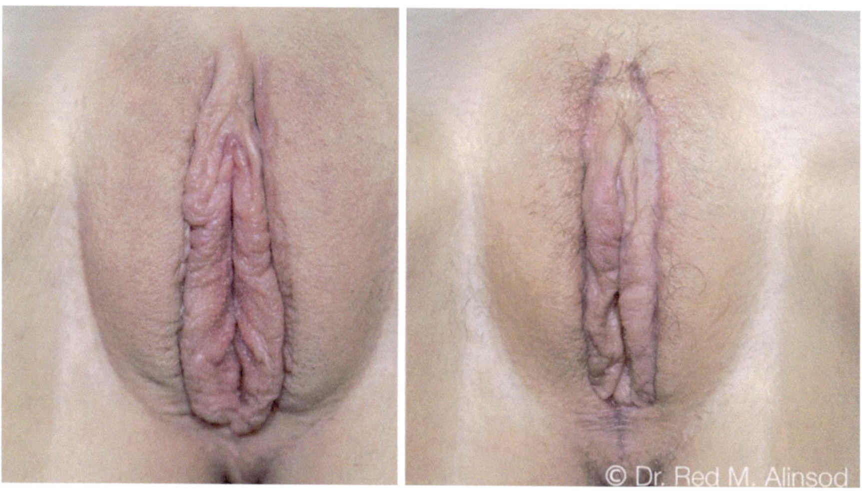

Fig. 11.21 Visible scars on the left photo. Scars hidden on the right photo

11.9 Scalloping of Surgical Edges

Scalloping of the labial edges is primarily a technical issue, often caused by overly tight suturing, excessive suture caliber, or inadequate postoperative care. Tying sutures too tightly can lead to "stair-stepping" of the incision edges, resulting in an irregular contour. To prevent this, surgeons should use "granny" or "air knots," avoid sutures larger than 4–0 Vicryl, and reinforce the importance of postoperative icing. Any remaining skin sutures should be removed at the 2-week postoperative visit to promote optimal healing and prevent unwanted contour irregularities. Surgeons should avoid external running or locking sutures, as these techniques can create unnecessary tension, contributing to scalloping and uneven wound healing. Instead, loosely tied interrupted sutures should be used on the surface of the labia majora, ensuring they provide adequate approximation without excessive tightness. Here is an example below of scalloping that has been eliminated with RF feathering in Figs. 11.22 and 11.23.

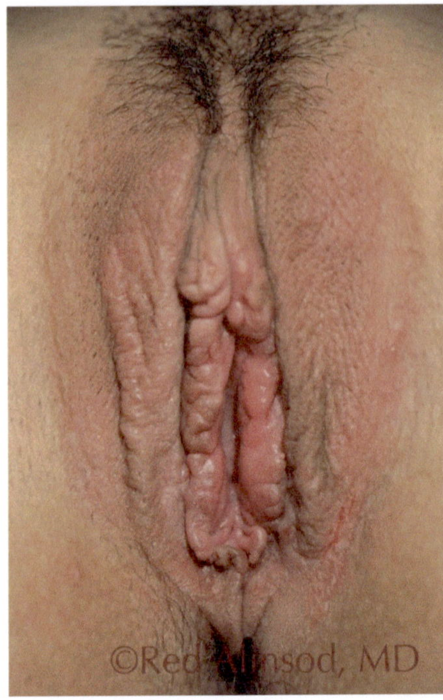

Fig. 11.22 Scalloping of suture lines

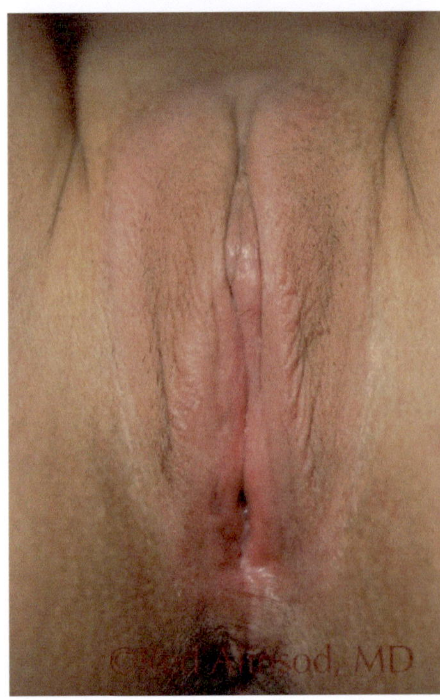

Fig. 11.23 RF feathering completed

11.10 Hypersensitivity of the Suture Line

Transient pudendal neuralgia or hypersensitivity of the suture line is a rare but distressing complication. Managing patient expectations through preoperative counseling is essential, as this condition is temporary and self-limiting. Treatment options include systemic medications such as pregabalin or gabapentin, although these may be associated with unwanted side effects. A preferable alternative is the application of local estrogen cream, which can be massaged into the suture line for at least 90 seconds once or twice daily to alleviate discomfort. Dr. Reed and Dr. Alinsod recommend a postoperative regimen that includes the nightly application of estrogen cream to the external surgical site to aid in tissue recovery and nerve desensitization. In the morning, a collagen and exosome cream are applied to further promote healing, reduce inflammation, and enhance overall comfort. This dual-therapy approach is advised for at least 4–6 weeks following surgery to optimize wound healing and minimize hypersensitivity.

11.11 Prominent Scar Formation and Keloids

While hypertrophic scarring and keloid formation are uncommon in labia majoraplasty, they can significantly impact both aesthetic and functional outcomes. Keloids result from an unchecked wound healing response, leading to excessive collagen deposition and progressive growth. Over the past 20 years, Dr. Alinsod has not encountered keloid formation following labia majoraplasty. In cosmetic gynecology, keloids are more commonly observed at the suture sites of clitoral hood reduction procedures rather than on the labia majora. These lesions do not resolve spontaneously and require active intervention. Intralesional corticosteroid injections, particularly with triamcinolone acetonide, are the most widely used treatment. Response rates vary, with 50–100% regression reported; however, recurrence remains a concern, occurring in 33% of cases after 1 year and 50% after 5 years [3]. Here is an example of early scar formation at the clitoral hood region. In this case, estrogen cream and massage softened the area, and normal appearance was restored, as seen in Figs. 11.24 and 11.25.

In this case below, a labia majoraplasty was performed and a firm scar formed at the clitoral hood suture site. This was resolved with one injection of Kenalog (Figs. 11.26, 11.27, and 11.28).

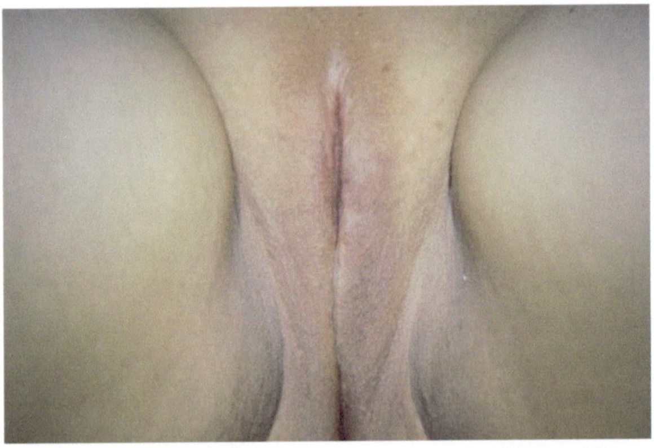

Fig. 11.24 Prominent scar on at the top

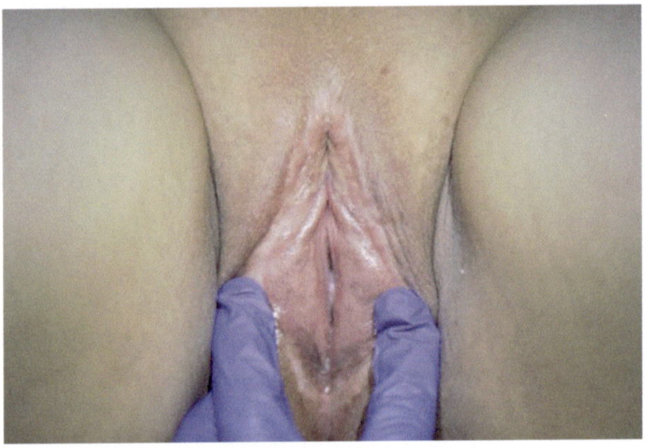

Fig. 11.25 After estrogen cream and massage

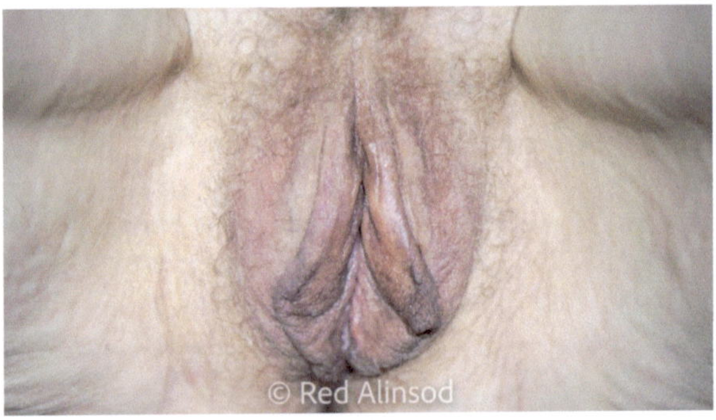

Fig. 11.26 Before surgery

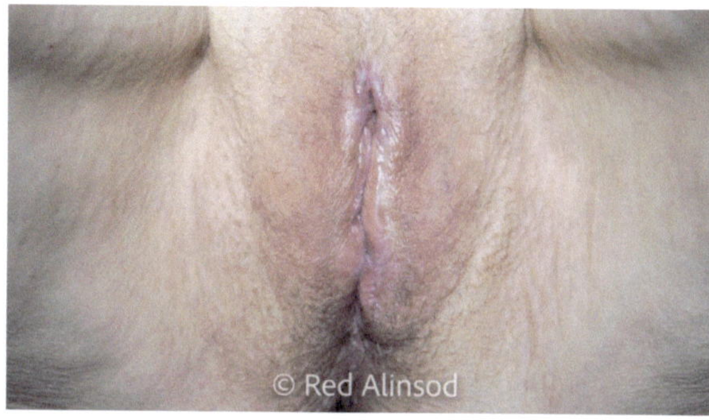

Fig. 11.27 Keloid before

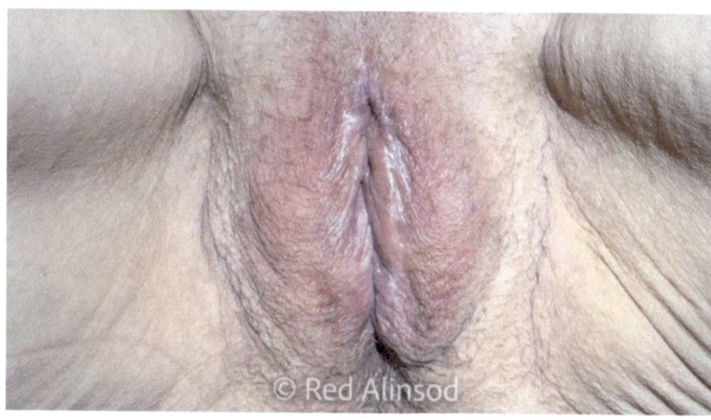

Fig. 11.28 After steroid

11.12 Gaping Introitus (Fish Mouth Appearance)

A gaping introitus or "fish mouth" deformity can occur if excessive labia majora tissue is excised, leading to lateral tension that pulls open the vestibule as shown in Figs. 11.29 and 11.30. This complication is best prevented through meticulous preoperative planning and intraoperative precision. The key to avoiding over-resection is to define the lateral extent of the excision within the natural ridge of the labia majora, preserving the apex and preventing excessive lateral pull.

To maintain natural contours, surgical markings should be carefully drawn preoperatively, ensuring that excision remains within the "top of the ridge," which represents the highest point of the labia majora. Avoiding excision beyond this anatomical boundary helps prevent unintended widening of the vaginal introitus. When necessary, combining a modest excision with volume restoration techniques can achieve a more balanced aesthetic while maintaining functional integrity. Patient counseling should also include discussions about this potential outcome to ensure informed consent and realistic postoperative expectations.

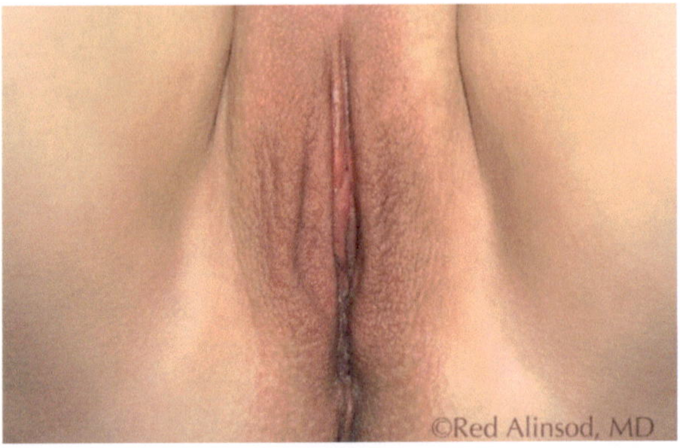

Fig. 11.29 Before surgery

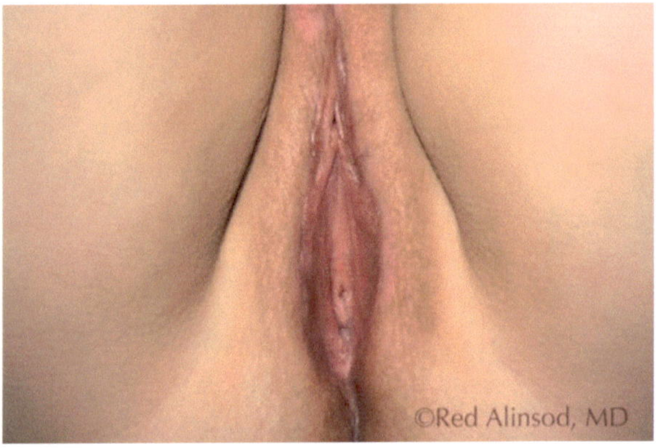

Fig. 11.30 After surgery with "Fish Mouth"

11.13 Infection: Urinary Tract Infections and Cellulitis

Routine antibiotic prophylaxis is not necessary for labia majoraplasty, as the risk of postoperative infection is low (less than 1% in Dr. Alinsod's 20-year series). However, in cases where there is instrumentation or manipulation near the urethra—such as sling procedures, anterior repairs, intravaginal RF or laser treatments, or catheterization—there is an increased risk of ascending infections. In these instances, patients may develop urinary tract infections (UTIs) or localized cellulitis, necessitating antibiotic therapy. First-line treatment options include macrodantin, cephalosporins, or penicillin-based agents such as amoxicillin-clavulanate (Augmentin) [2]. Close monitoring for early signs of infection ensures timely intervention and prevents complications from progressing.

11.14 Constipation from Narcotic Use

Postoperative constipation is a frequent issue, often exacerbated by opioid analgesics. Prevention starts with adequate hydration and dietary modifications, including increased intake of dried prunes (8–10 per day) or cold prune juice. Over-the-counter stool softeners, such as docusate sodium, can be used twice daily. Milk of magnesia works quite well to reduce this problem when narcotics are being taken early on. If constipation persists beyond 3 days, stronger interventions like senna-based laxatives, polyethylene glycol (Miralax), or herbal teas such as "Smooth Move" may be necessary [3].

11.15 Pubic Hair in the Suture Line Crease

In some patients, pubic hair growth extends into the crease between the labia minora and labia majora, potentially causing irritation along the suture line. This issue is typically not problematic for individuals who routinely shave or wax their vulvar region. For those seeking a long-term solution, laser hair reduction or intense pulsed light (IPL) treatments can effectively manage hair growth in this area, improving patient comfort [4].

11.16 Conclusion

Recognizing and managing complications after labia majoraplasty is essential for ensuring patient satisfaction and optimal surgical outcomes. While most postoperative issues are minor and self-limiting, early identification and appropriate intervention can prevent more serious complications. A combination of meticulous surgical technique, thorough patient education, and proactive postoperative care allows for the best possible recovery experience. With an emphasis on prevention and patient-centered management, labia majoraplasty can be performed safely and effectively, minimizing risks while maximizing aesthetic and functional benefits.

Disclosure The authors of this chapter have no commercial or financial conflicts.

References

1. Morelli Coppola M, Salzillo R, Segreto F, Persichetti P. Triamcinolone acetonide intralesional injection for the treatment of keloid scars: patient selection and perspectives. Clin Cosmet Investig Dermatol. 2018;11:387–96.
2. Van Le L, Handa VL, Patterson D, editors. Te Linde's operative gynecology. 13th ed. Philadelphia: Lippincott Williams & Wilkins; 2024.
3. Stolecka-Warzecha A, Chmielewski Ł, Deda A, Smich P, Wawrzynek W. Experimental research of the pharmacological. J Orthop Case Rep. 2023;13(12):11–7.
4. Hamori C, Banwell PE, Alinsod RM. Female cosmetic genital surgery. Thieme; 2017.

Chapter 12
What Comes After Labia Majora Treatments

Pablo Gonzalez Isaza

Any treatment for aesthetic and functional reasons in labia majora should have a standardized follow-up and after care to ensure optimal results.

As a part of our algorithmic approach, we always consider crucial to have defined time intervals for touch-up sessions, when we are using either energy-based devices, fillers, threads, or collagen bio-stimulators.

For more severe cases there is always the need, either to perform a labia majora labiaplasty or to use strategies that follow the principles of combined bio-stimulation (Table 12.1).

Immediately after a labia majora labiaplasty, we ask our patients to follow basic principles of wound care, such as intermittent ice, compression, garments with ozonized oil, analgesics, and hygiene, after about 7–10 days usually after suture material is removed or absorbed, we perform infrared light blue color 417 nm sessions to speed up healing and improve inflammation, and once the healing process is completed, our patients are scheduled for touch-up sessions according to the clinical situation, among our options are fractional Co_2 laser, preferred for skin rejuvenation and pigmentation.

We also have available different types of bipolar radiofrequency-based platforms for skin laxity and adipose atrophy conditions (Fig. 12.1); intervals for planned touch-up sessions will be scheduled immediately after the surgical procedure.

After ablative procedures in labia majora (laser or fractional needle radiofrequency is performed), our nurses apply an alginate-based mask with special components to reduce inflammation and speed up healing time (Fig. 12.2).

When hyaluronic acid-based fillers or collagen bio-stimulators such as calcium hydroxyapatite and polylactic acid were used as a combined strategy during the first

P. Gonzalez Isaza (✉)
Obstetrics and Gynecology, Urogynecology Minimally Invasive Surgery, Hospital Universitario San Jorge, Pereira, Colombia

Soranus Center for Funtional and Regenerative Urogynecology, Pereira, Colombia

P. Gonzalez Isaza (ed.), *Aesthetic and Functional Alterations of the Labia Majora*, https://doi.org/10.1007/978-3-031-97405-2_12

Table 12.1 Combined of treatments for labia majora aesthetic and functional complaints

Cutaneous Hyperlaxity (CHL) MILD	Adipose Hypertrophy (AH)	Cutaneous Adipose Atrophy (CAA)	Iatrogenic Conditions (IC)
External RF (multipolar, monopolar) Fractional CO_2 laser Erbium Yag laser	Liposuction Lipectomy (rule out site-specific defects with deep fat sac protrusion) Fractional Combinations Consider microneedle ablative RF	Fillers hyaluronic acid Fat grafting PRP Combinations	Hyaluronic acid Hyaluronidase/collagenase injections Labiaplasty Combinations Fat Laser lipolysis Lipectomy (rule out site-specific defects with deep fat sac protrusion) Intracavitary RF Permanent fillers Laser lipolysis Lipectomy Combinations
Laxity/tone (LT) Moderate			
Microneedle ablative RF			
Intracavitary RF			
PDO-PLLA-PCL (suspension bio-stimulation threads) Combinations			
Labiapexy			
Laxity/tone (LT) Severe			
Labiaplasty site-specific repairs			
Lipectomy			
Combinations			

surgical procedure, patients are also scheduled for touch-up sessions according to the clinical effect of the products, usually crosslinked hyaluronic acid-based fillers will remain in average 9–14 months depending on the patients activities, and regarding collagen bio-stimulators, the main effect will be dependent on the degree of collagen stimulation of the patient, in average 18–24 months.

Another important aspect to consider after any labia majora treatment is the hair removal method, razors, creams, and waxing are related to skin pigmentation, which could be an aesthetic complaint, and in our center as a part of the protocol for labia majora enhancing we offer safe laser-based hair removal with a special device that has a hybrid wavelength (alexandrite 655 nm and Nd-Yag 1064 nm); this feature offers excellent results and efficacy, avoiding hyperpigmentation, Fig. 12.3.

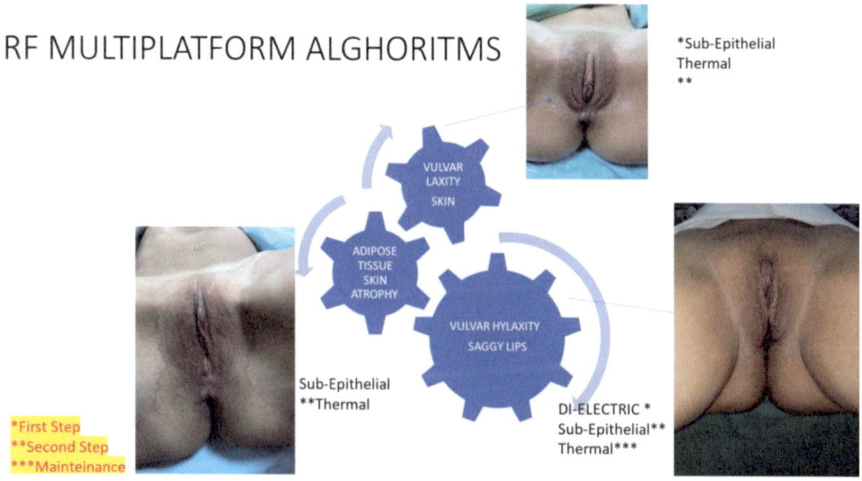

Fig. 12.1 Labia majora aesthetic and functional alterations approach with multimodal radiofrequency platform. Different types of Radiofrequency are used according to the clinical situation of the patient, for severe cases of atrophy and skin aging, non-ablative thermal radiofrequency is preferred, and in contrast for cases of skin laxity in younger patients, fractional ablative radiofrequency is preferred

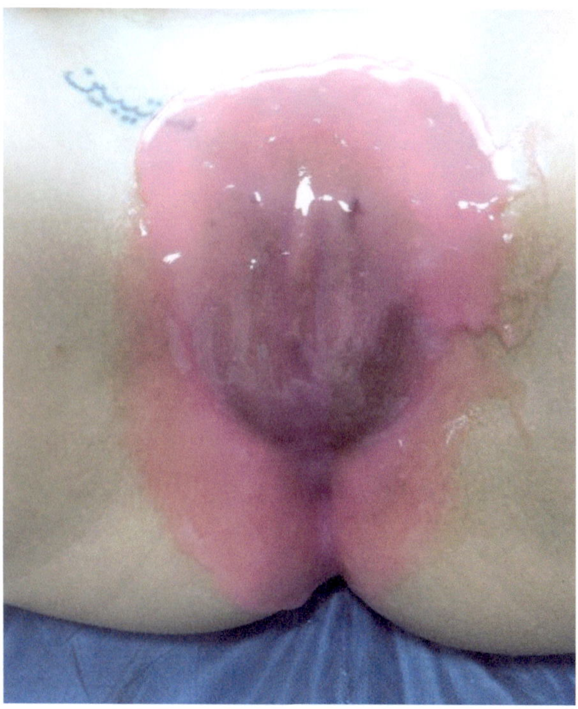

Fig. 12.2 Alginate-based mask after ablative procedures in labia majora

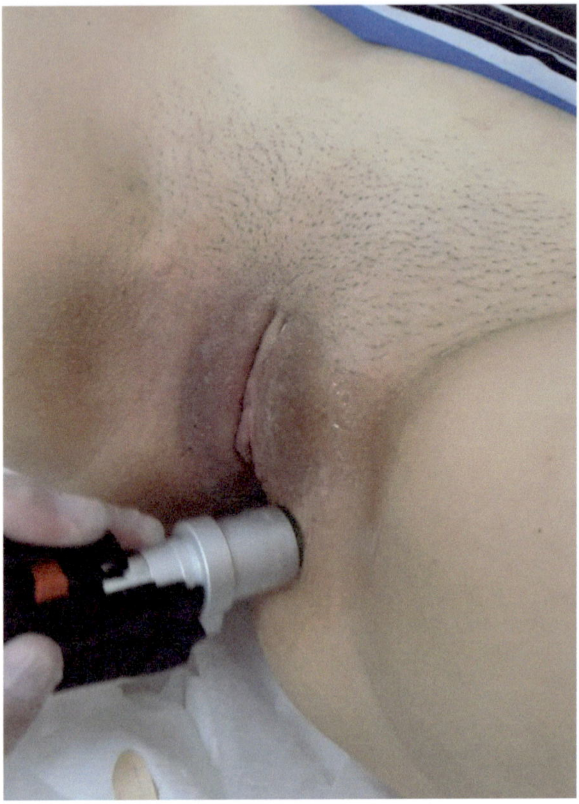

Fig. 12.3 Laser hair removal (hybrid wavelength to improve and avoid pigmentation)

Reference

1. DeMaria AL, Flores M, Hirth JM, Berenson AB. Complications related to pubic hair removal. Am J Obstet Gynecol. 2014;210(6):528.e1–5. https://doi.org/10.1016/j.ajog.2014.01.036. Epub 2014 Jan 31. PMID: 24486227; PMCID: PMC4040320.

Chapter 13
Sexological Impact

Diana Lorena Vélez Rizo

Female identity and self-esteem is closely related to genital self-perception. The practice of hair removal and self-examination has led to greater awareness of the intimate area and with it the search for procedures to improve the appearance of the genital area [1, 2].

Women seek a regenerative and functional aesthetic gynecology procedure not only for aesthetic but also for functional purposes, and this search may be related to the desire to improve their sexual satisfaction and, secondarily, an increase in self-esteem by changing genital perception, improving security and self-image [3].

Labiaplasty of the labia majora is a safe procedure with a positive impact on multiple areas of a woman's life.

Labia majora have a highly erotic component, so sexual dissatisfaction and sexual discomfort are reasons for requesting labiaplasty. These women report increased anxiety when their partner sees or touches their genitals, as well as fear that they will no longer be attractive and that their encounters will cease [1, 2].

At a psychosocial level, labia majora are affected by different factors such as age, weight loss, etc. Woman may perceive genital abnormality, negatively affecting

D. L. V. Rizo (✉)
Gynecologist and Obstetrician Universidad de la Sabana, Cundinamarca, Colombia

Colposcopy and Cervical Pathology Universidad Nacional de, Bogotá, Colombia

Laser and Gynecologic Functional Aesthetic Surgery AGEOC Association of Colombian Aesthetic Gynecologists, Bogotá, Colombia

Laser applications in gynecology Universidad Nacional de, Bogotá, Colombia

Master in Clinical Sexology, University of Valencia, Valencia, Spain

Urological and Reconstructive Gynecology of the Pelvic Floor National University of Colombia, Bogotá, Colombia

Gynecologist in Dr. Diana Velez Rizo Advanced Gynecology, Fundación Cardioinfantil and Clínica de la Mujer, Bogotá, Colombia

P. Gonzalez Isaza (ed.), *Aesthetic and Functional Alterations of the Labia Majora*, https://doi.org/10.1007/978-3-031-97405-2_13

sexual self-esteem, and volume depletion may translate into a functional problem by drying out and exposing the labia minora and vaginal introitus.

Labia majora fulfill different functions, including allowing the direction and entry of sperm into the body, protecting the genital organs from infectious agents, and maintaining lubrication and sexual pleasure during sexual intercourse [3].

Sexually, ptosis of the Mons Venus and labia majora can make access to clitoral areas difficult, and, although it is not directly related as a cause of sexual dysfunction, it can cause symptoms of low satisfaction. Such procedures can be challenging but are highly successful under trained hands, leading to markedly improved self-image and quality of life along with a return of satisfactory sexual activity and elimination of discomfort [4].

The clitoral hood, and the clitoris itself, is one of the most sensitive areas on a sexual level. During genital aesthetic surgery, it is appropriate to pay attention to preserving the integrity of the skin flap in this area; for this reason the midline should be preserved, and the labia majora incisions should not join together [5].

It has been demonstrated by magnetic resonance imaging of the genital organs during arousal that the labia majora do not present changes in size or enhancement, but the vulva is the largest exposed structure and therefore the most visible [6].

Reconstruction of the labia majora also allows for improved sensitivity in the midline, mainly when iatrogenic amputations have occurred by limiting the exposure of areas that normally should not be exposed. Furthermore, positive genital image has been shown to improve general sexual desire in Female Sexual Function Index FSFI [7, 8].

In a trial of 217 women, an online survey was applied where they evaluated the body image in the context of sexuality, focusing on two very specific dimensions: satisfaction with the visual appearance of the genitals and shyness about the genitals during a sexual encounter. The analysis revealed that greater dissatisfaction with genital appearance was associated with greater self-awareness of genital image during intimacy and was associated with lower self-esteem, sexual satisfaction, and motivation to avoid risky sexual behaviors. These findings underscore the detrimental impact of negative genital perceptions on women's sexual well-being. Interventions that improve satisfaction with the natural appearance of your genitals could facilitate the development of a healthy sexual self-concept and provide long-term benefits in terms of sexual confidence and satisfaction [9].

Within the clinical history, risk factors that require multidisciplinary management with sexology, psychology, and/or psychiatry should be evaluated, such as women who have been victims of sexual abuse, those who have suffered negative comments about their genitals, or patients with a high probability of body dysmorphic syndrome [10].

Body dysmorphic syndrome is identified in 7–13% of people seeking aesthetic treatments and should be suspected preoperatively when there is an excessive preoccupation with a defect of mild or unobservable appearance that is associated with obsessive thinking, and compulsive behaviors that lead to impact daily living activities diagnostic criteria are established by DSM-V [11].

Body dysmorphic syndrome is treatable and a relative contraindication to taking the patient to surgery if it has not been treated, but with a good response to cognitive behavioral or pharmacological management of up to 84.6% [10].

What scales can we use to evaluate patients?

The use of validated instruments in preoperative evaluations to assess the level of discomfort regarding physical appearance and satisfaction helps in patient selection despite the fact that there is no specific scale for the evaluation of the labia majora [12].

The most widely used is the validated GAS (*Genital Appearance Satisfaction*) scale, which has 11 items on attitudes toward genital appearance. Each item is scored between 0 and 3 (from "Never" to "Always") with total scores between 0 and 33. The higher the score is, the greater the genital dissatisfaction [13].

The COPS-L scale (Cosmetic Procedure Screening Scale modified for labia) focuses on concerns about the appearance of the lips and is derived from the COPS (Cosmetic Procedure Screening Scale) that assesses overall appearance. COPS-L focuses on the domains of perceived abnormality, effect on sexual intercourse, interference with leisure activities, conspicuousness in public, and comparison with others. The questionnaire is answered according to a Likert scale that ranges from 0 to 8 for each of the questions. It is scored by adding all the elements to provide a total value calculation. Possible total scores range from 0 to 72. Scores above 40 reflect greater preoccupation, distress, and disability with a body characteristic and therefore the likelihood of a body dysmorphic syndrome diagnosis [12].

The FSFI scale was described by Rosen in 2000, and it is a 19-item questionnaire with psychometric properties designed to be an instrument for the assessment of female sexual function. It is used to measure sexual function in heterosexual women who have been sexually active in the past 4 weeks. The questions are answered on a *Likert* scale ranging from 0 to 5 or from 1 to 5 depending on the item and include a total of six factors (Desire, Arousal, Lubrication, Orgasm, Satisfaction, and Pain). Total scores less than or equal to 26 indicate the presence of sexual dysfunction [14, 15].

Assessing the presence of *female sexual dysfunction* and *body dysmorphic syndrome* with the FSFI and COPS-L scales, respectively, helps to guide medical decisions and the patient in order to clarify expectations, raise awareness, educate, and guide patients.

References

1. Sahin F, Mihmanli V. The impact of labiaplasty on sexuality. Ginekol Pol. 2024;95(8):596–600. https://doi.org/10.5603/gpl.94975. Epub 2023 Dec 15. PMID: 38099665.
2. Laan E, Martoredjo DK, Hesselink S, Snijders N, van Lunsen RHW. Young women's genital self-image and effects of exposure to pictures of natural vulvas. J Psychosom Obstet Gynaecol. 2017;38(4):249–55. https://doi.org/10.1080/0167482X.2016.1233172. Epub 2016 Sep 20. PMID: 27649469.

3. Salgado CJ, Tang JC, Desrosiers AE 3rd. Use of dermal fat graft for augmentation of the labia majora. J Plast Reconstr Aesthet Surg. 2012;65(2):267–70. https://doi.org/10.1016/j.bjps.2011.07.010. Epub 2011 Jul 30
4. Alter GJ. Pubic contouring after massive weight loss in men and women: correction of hidden penis, Mons ptosis, and labia majora enlargement. Plast Reconstr Surg. 2012;130(4):936–47. https://doi.org/10.1097/PRS.0b013e318262f57d.
5. Schober JM, Meyer-Bahlburg HF, Ransley PG. Self-assessment of genital anatomy, sexual sensitivity and function in women: implications for genitoplasty. BJU Int. 2004;94(4):589–94. https://doi.org/10.1111/j.1464-410X.2004.05006.x. PMID: 15329118.
6. Suh DD, Yang CC, Cao Y, Heiman JR, Garland PA, Maravilla KR. MRI of female genital and pelvic organs during sexual arousal. J Psychosom Obstet Gynaecol. 2004;25(2):153–62. https://doi.org/10.1080/01674820400002220. PMID: 15715038.
7. Vogt PM, Herold C, Rennekampff HO. Autologous fat transplantation for labia majora reconstruction. Aesth Plast Surg. 2011;35(5):913–5. https://doi.org/10.1007/s00266-011-9664-5. Epub 2011 Feb 27. PMID: 21359987.
8. Berman L, Berman J, Miles M, Pollets D, Powell JA. Genital self-image as a component of sexual health: relationship between genital self-image, female sexual function, and quality of life measures. J Sex Marital Ther. 2003;29(Suppl 1):11–21. https://doi.org/10.1080/713847124.
9. Schick VR, Calabrese SK, Rima BN, Zucker AN. Genital appearance dissatisfaction: implications for women's genital image self-consciousness, Sexual esteem, Sexual satisfaction, and Sexual risk. Psychol Women Q. 2010;34(3):394–404. https://doi.org/10.1111/j.1471-6402.2010.01584.x. PMID: 20824180; PMCID: PMC2931365
10. Müllerová J, Weiss P. Plastic surgery in gynaecology: factors affecting women's decision to undergo labiaplasty. Mind the risk of body dysmorphic disorder: a review. J Women Aging. 2020;32(3):241–58. https://doi.org/10.1080/08952841.2018.1529474.
11. Sarwer DB. Body image, cosmetic surgery, and minimally invasive treatments. Body Image. 2019;31:302–8. https://doi.org/10.1016/j.bodyim.2019.01.009.
12. De Brito MJA, Nahas FX, Sabino NM. Invited response on: body dysmorphic disorder: is there an "ideal" strategy? Aesth Plast Surg. 2019;43(4):1115–6. https://doi.org/10.1007/s00266-019-01384-8.
13. Veale D, Eshkevari E, Ellison N, Cardozo L, Robinson D, Kavouni A. Validation of genital appearance satisfaction scale and the cosmetic procedure screening scale for women seeking labiaplasty. J Psychosom Obstet Gynaecol. 2013;34(1):46–52. https://doi.org/10.3109/0167482X.2012.756865.
14. Vallejo-Medina P, Pérez-Durán C, Saavedra-Roa A. Translation, adaptation, and preliminary Validation of the female Sexual function Index into Spanish (Colombia). Arch Sex Behav. 2018;47(3):797–810.
15. Validation P, Sexual F, Index F, Behavior S. 1.2 validated version in Colombia of the female Sexual function Index. (FSFI; Rosen et al., 2000), vol. 61; 2017.

Chapter 14
Fat Grafting of Labia Majora from Theory to Clinical Practice

Pablo Gonzalez Isaza and Gustavo Leibaschoff

14.1 Introduction

Subcutaneous fat tissue has been in use for many years for correction and remodeling purposes. The first use of autologous fat transplantation was described by Neuber in 1893 [1], by filling small soft tissue defects. Regarding female body, Czerny in 1895 reported the use of free fat graft, for complete reconstruction of breast defects [1]. The first reports of autologous fat transplantations to the genital tract followed the principles of Coleman technique regarding aspiration, harvesting and injection, posteriorly widely accepted for different indications in gynecology which were not only for aesthetic indications but also for functional aims [2]. It can be considered an invaluable tool because it is readily available, easy to harvest, has low morbidity, affordable, and biocompatible. Ya-Wei et al. in a recent study reported an important improvement of sexual functioning measured by FSFI questionnaire after autologous fat grafting; according to their findings it could be explained by the stimulation of estrogen receptors that lead to collagenesis and angionesis [3].

Among all the described procedures related to female genital cosmetic surgery, the option of labia majora enhancement or augmentation remains an everyday demand from our patients. Massive weight loss after bariatric surgery, chronic stretching from waxing, or just aging are the most common causes of labia majora laxity, and sometimes the demand for a combined labia minora labiaplasty procedure is performed.

P. Gonzalez Isaza (✉)
Obstetrics and Gynecology, Urogynecology Minimally invasive Surgery,
Hospital Universitario San Jorge, Pereira, Colombia

Soranus Center for Funtional and Regenerative Urogynecology, Pereira, Colombia

G. Leibaschoff
Obstetrician and Gynecologist Private Practice, Dallas, TX, USA
e-mail: drghl@icam-usa.com

P. Gonzalez Isaza (ed.), *Aesthetic and Functional Alterations of the Labia Majora*, https://doi.org/10.1007/978-3-031-97405-2_14

A female genital cosmetic surgeon must follow a structured technique, from a good selection of the donor area to the correct injection inside labia majora for aesthetic and functional purposes.

14.2 Labia Majora Augmentation

14.2.1 Technique

Our experience in female genital cosmetic procedures regarding fat grafting started in 2010 when we traveled to Buenos Aires Argentina to meet Professor Gustavo Leibaschoff, a world renowned female cosmetic genital surgeon with great knowledge of adipose tissue, and we learned a very structured technique to harvest and inject fat in labia majora with great results (Table 14.1). A good selection of the donor area is crucial for fat survival, and also higher concentration of adipose-derived stem cells (ADSCs) is found in the lower abdomen and inner thigh [4].

Patients are under sedation. A modified Klein solution is of our preference to avoid the use of lidocaine inside because it has been demonstrated to affect adipocyte function, due to lipolysis and glucose transport. Lidocaine inside tumescent solution can also increase fibrosis and necrosis [5]. Our preparation keeps all the other components of Klein's solution, such as normal saline solution, adrenaline, and bicarbonate (Table 14.1).

Skin incisions are performed with a # 11 scalpel in areas where scars are not easily noticeable, then tumescent solution is injected, and after 10 minutes aspiration is performed using a 2.0-mm Tonnard cannula and 10-mL Luer-Lok syringes using low negative pressure (Fig. 14.1); normally the aspiration ratio is 1–1, and the total volume aspirated is around 100–200 cc according to the clinical conditions and needs of our patients.

Table 14.1 Structured technique for labia majora fat grafting, AGEOC Clinical Practice Guidelines 2025

Tumescent solution	Donor site	Aspiration technique	Harvesting and processing	Injection
1000 cc normal saline 1 CC adrenaline 12.5 mEq sodium bicarbonate	Lower abdomen Pubis Inner thigh	2 mm cannulas Low pressure 10 cc syringes	Washing with normal saline and decantation	1–2 mm cannula retrograde multiplane technique

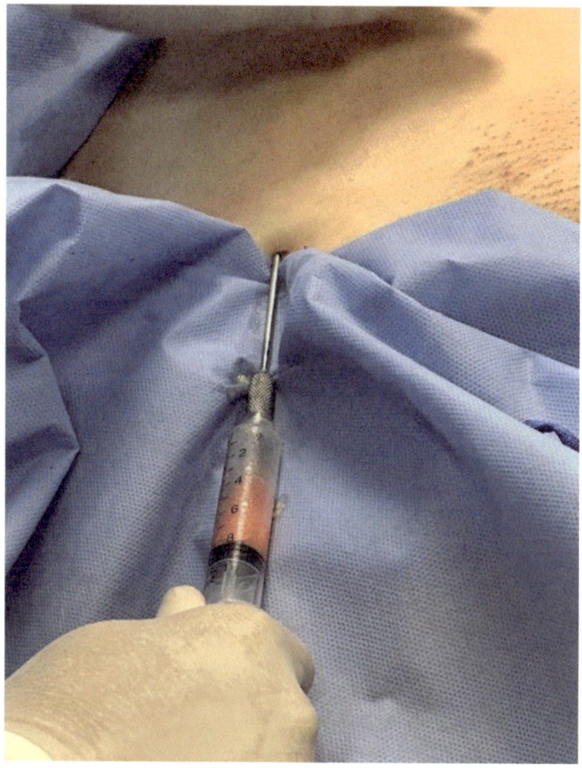

Fig. 14.1 Technique of aspiration suprapubic fat. (Dr. Pablo Gonzalez Isaza, personal archive)

After aspiration fat is later separated by traditional decantation technique, for 3–5 minutes, afterward, all remnants from infiltration are removed (Fig. 14.2). The use of centrifuges is expensive, and evidence regarding adipocytes survival after the centrifugation process remains controversial [7].

Fat is injected with retrograde technique in a three-layer fashion under the dartos fascia following the principle of Eto et al. who state that survival of the regenerating zone is related to adipose-derived stromal cells (ASCs) responsible for the survival of the implant [6] (Figs. 14.3 and 14.4).

The preparation of nano fat is a specialized process that involves the use of a kit of filters from 2000 to 500 microns to obtain the product rich in adipose-derived stromal cells (ASCs) that will be injected intradermally to enhance the regenerating zone. (Fig. 14.6 and 14.7).

There are multiple options in the market for nano fat processing; some of them are expensive and not easily available inside some countries (Table 14.2).

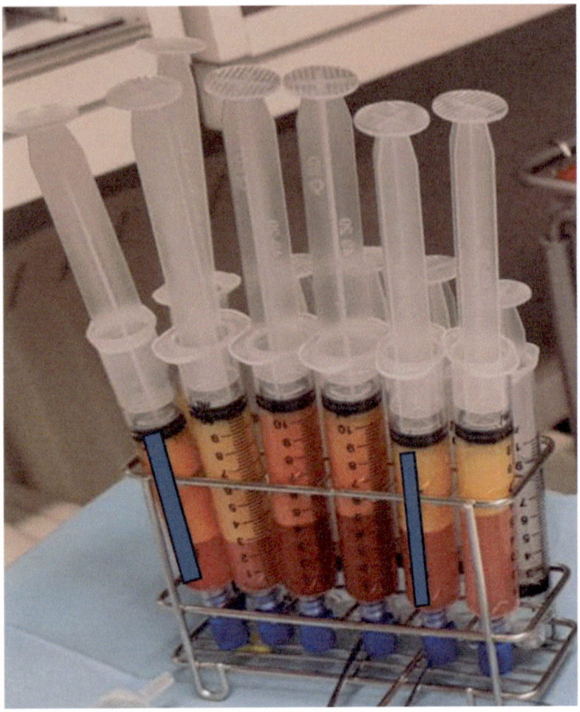

Fig. 14.2 Fat washing and decantation. (Dr. Pablo Gonzalez Isaza, personal archive)

Plasma-rich platelet after centrifugation at 2000 rpm for 10 min is added in a proportion of 2 cc per each 10 cc of fat; the rationale for this approach is to enhance the survival of adipocytes due to the release of growth factors and exosomes [8].

After the fat is injected, a gentle massage is performed to have a more homogeneous implant, and patients are discharged home with clear post-op recommendations.

Besides labia majora volume enhancement, fat grafting is usually performed as a combined procedure for other indications such as botched labiaplasties, due to the increase of complications of labia minora approach by untrained surgeons.; sometimes it is not possible to perform flaps and other reconstructive techniques due to the type of amputation performed [8] (Figs. 14.8 and 14.9, 14.10 and 14.11).

Vogt et al. performed successful labia majora fat grafting after vulvectomy due to malignant conditions and surgical trauma, and this approach offers not only anatomical restoration but also a better quality of life [9].

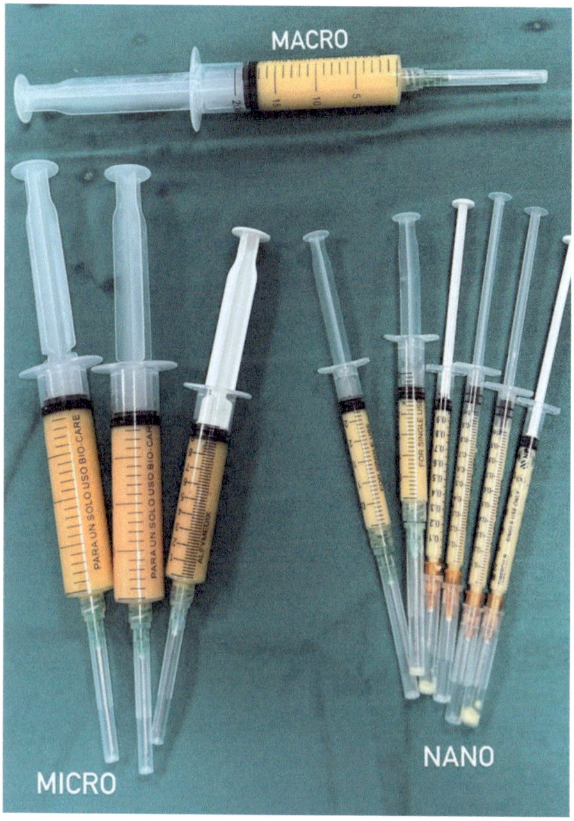

Fig. 14.3 Lipoaspirate after washing and decantation. (Dr. Pablo Gonzalez Isaza, personal archive)

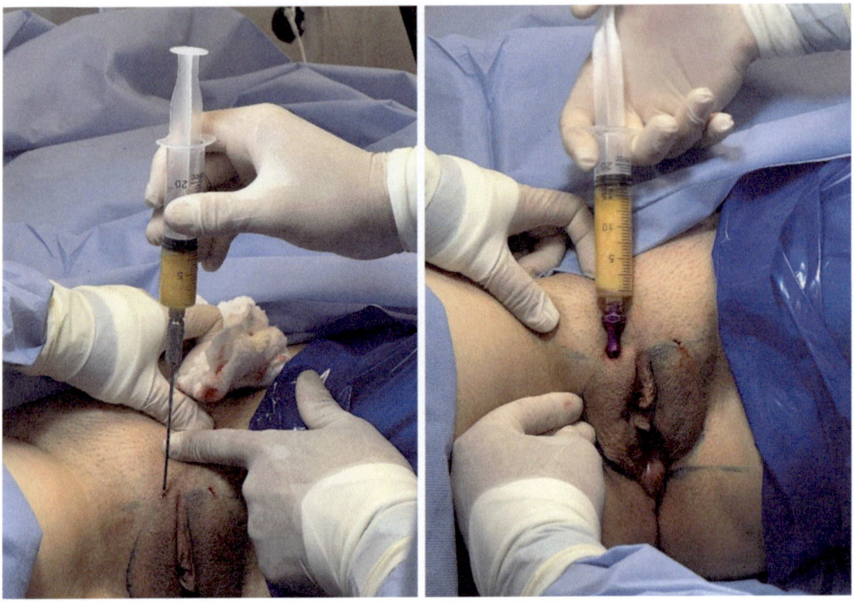

Figs. 14.4 and 14.5 Technique for fat graft injection into labia majora. (Dr. Pablo Gonzalez Isaza, personal archive)

Fig. 14.6 Nano fat filters kit. (Dr. Pablo Gonzalez Isaza, personal archive)

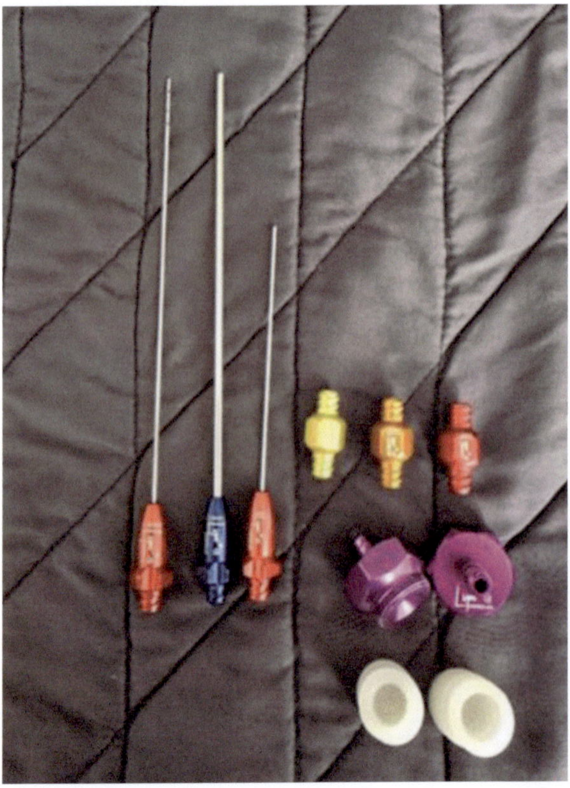

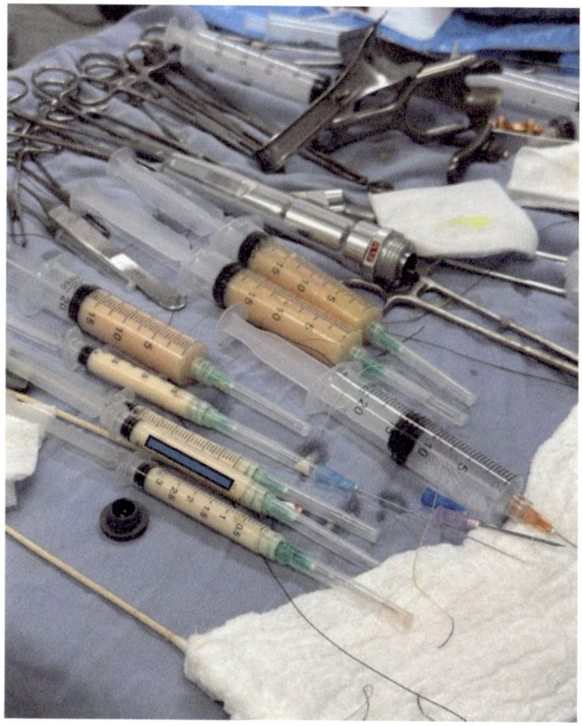

Fig. 14.7 Nano fat processing. (Dr. Pablo Gonzalez Isaza, personal archive)

Table 14.2 Different options and terminology for adipose-derived stromal cells (ASCs) processing

Tool	Brand	Filters	Centrifugue	Canula needle	Injection plane	Regeneration	Anti inflammatory effect	Volumizing effect
Ultra nanofat exosomes	–	80 microns	NO	32/34	Intradermal	+	+++	No
Nano fat	FIDIA	120 microns	NO	30	Subdermal	++	++	+
Nano fat	Nano cube	400 microns	NO	27	Subdermal	++	++	++
Nano fat	Filters	600 microns	NO	25	Subdermal	++	++	++
Nano fat	Filters	900 microns	Decantation	18/21	Dermal	++	++	+++
Nano fat	Filters	1000 microns	Decantation	18/21	Dermal	++	++	+++
Nano fat	Filters Lipocube	1500 microns	Decantation	18/21	Dermal	++	++	+++
PRP	–		YES 2000/8 MIN	34	Intradermal	+	+ +	No

AGEOC Clinical Practice Guidelines 2025

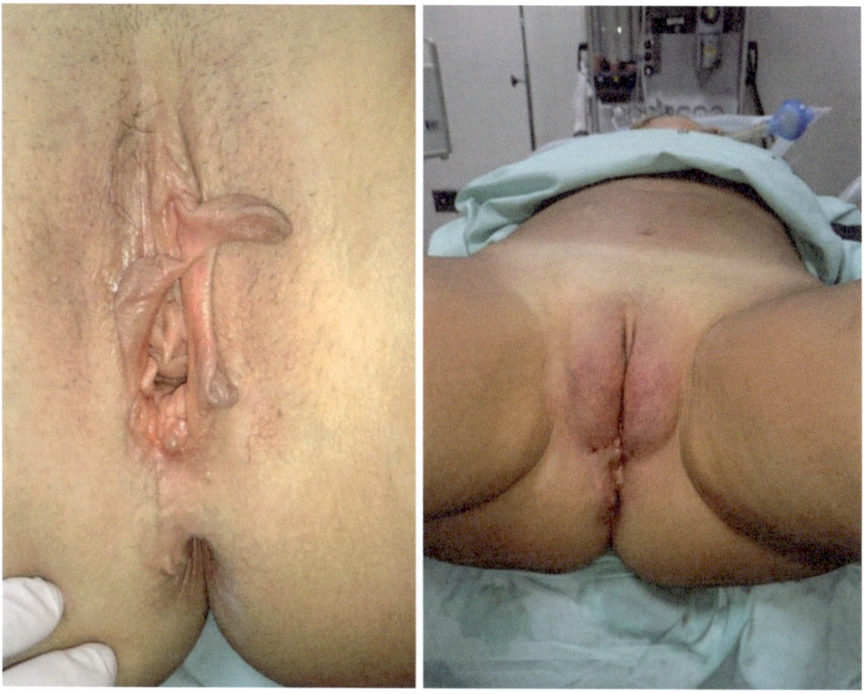

Figs. 14.8 and 14.9 Before and after reconstructive topographic CO_2 laser labiaplasty + autologous fat grafting. (Dr. Pablo Gonzalez Isaza, personal archive)

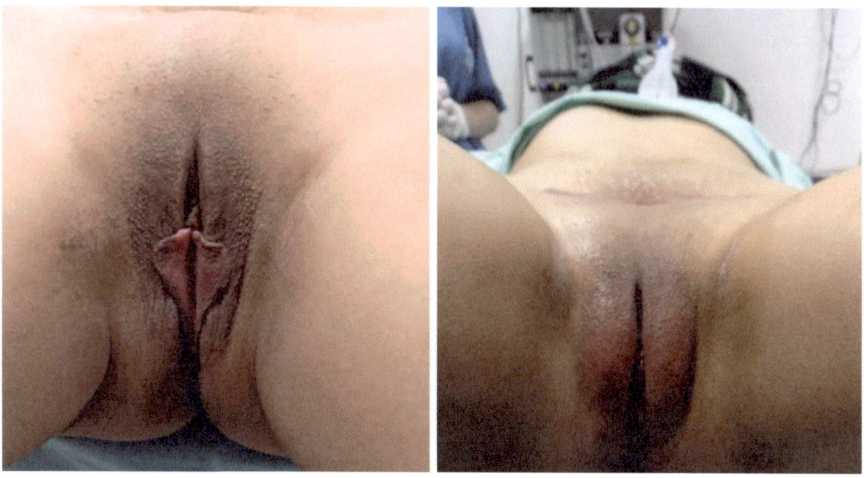

Figs. 14.10 and 14.11 Before and after labia minora CO_2 laser labiaplasty combined with labia majora autologous fat grafting. (Dr. Pablo Gonzalez Isaza, personal archive)

Table 14.3 Rate of complications of labia majora fat grafting inside our statistics

Granulomas 9%	Oil Cysts 0.9%	Hematomas 0.5%
Infections 0%	Fast absorption 30%	

AGEOC Clinical Practice Guidelines 2025

14.3 Complications

Autologous fat grafting for gynecological indications can be considered a safe treatment; hence complications are extremely rare but usually are described as the same for fat grafting, in body contouring procedures, such as hematomas, granulomas, fat necrosis, oil cyst formation, infection, and temporary pain (Table 14.3). A rare case of a woman who developed severe fat embolism after autologous fat grafting for vaginal tightening and breast augmentation surgery was described by Chenyu et al., and it was assumed to have occurred by injection of large volumes of fat directly into the vessels around the vagina. The patient survived after intensive care unit management.

14.4 Conclusions

Fat grafting for labia majora is a safe and efficient alternative invaluable tool in regenerative medicine and surgery highly accepted by patients. It can be performed for multiples indications: aesthetic, reconstructive, or functional, alone or in combination with other surgical techniques. It must be standardized inside female aesthetic genital surgery practitioners and should be performed by trained physicians, to achieve the best results and ensure patient safety [10].

14.5 Atlas of Images

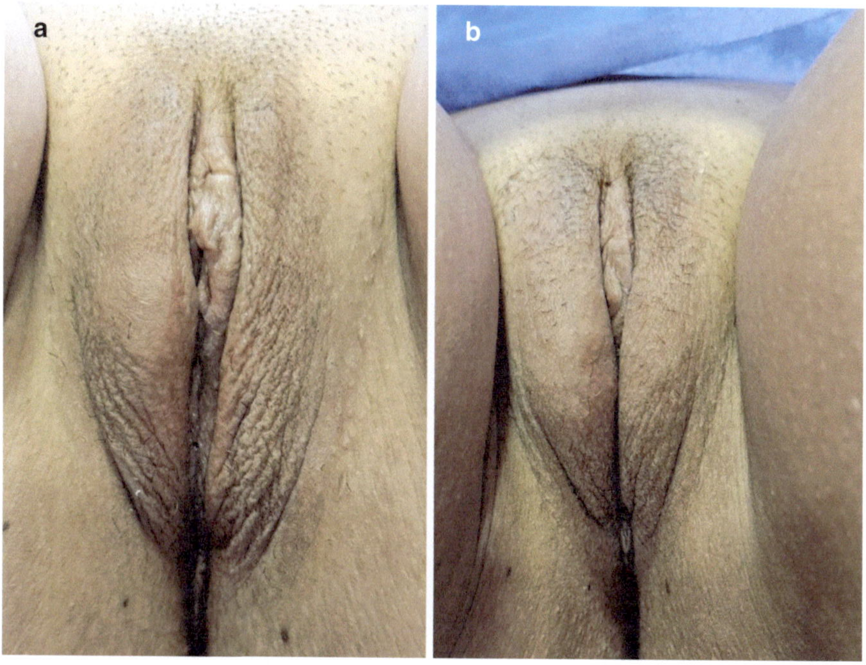

Fig. 14.12 (**a**, **b**) Before and after 6-month labia majora and autologous fat grafting. (Dr. Pablo Gonzalez Isaza, personal archive)

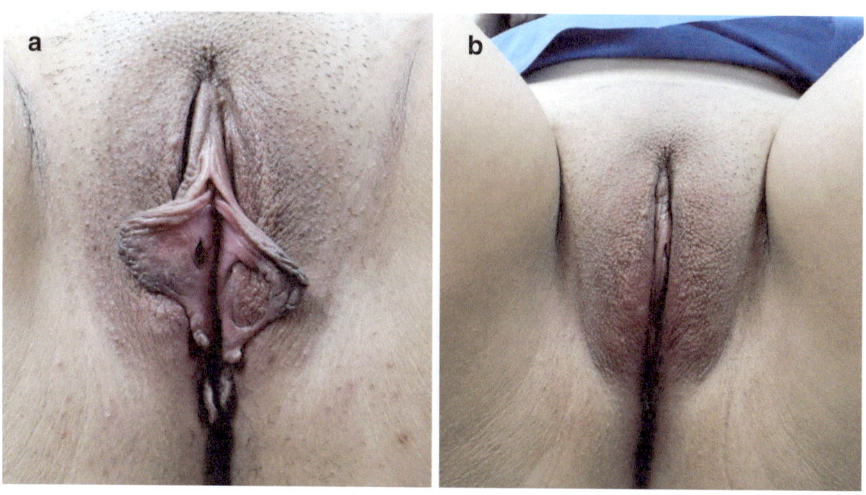

Fig. 14.13 (**a**, **b**) Before and after 1-month reconstructive topographic labiaplasty and autologous fat grafting. (Dr. Pablo Gonzalez Isaza, personal archive)

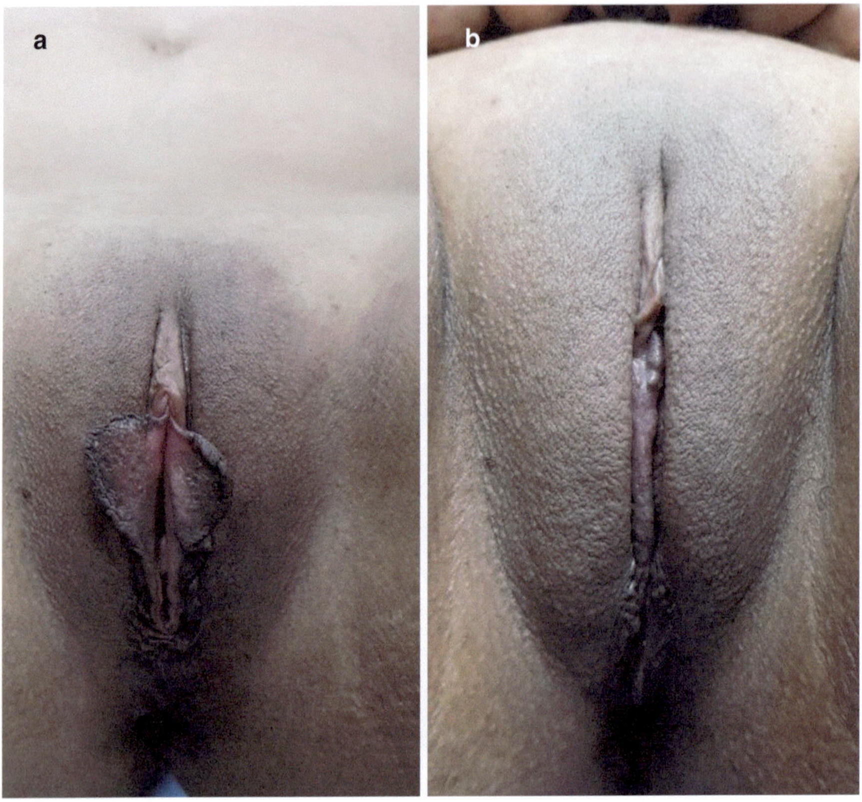

Fig. 14.14 (**a, b**) Before and after topographic labiaplasty and autologous fat grafting. (Dr. Pablo Gonzalez Isaza, personal archive)

References

1. Billings EJ, May JW Jr. Historical review and present status of free fat graft autotransplantation in plastic and reconstructive surgery. Plast Reconstr Surg. 1989;83(2):368–81.
2. Coleman SR. Facial recontouring with lipostructure. Clin Plast Surg. 1997;242:347–67.
3. Lai YW, Wu SH, Chou PR, Lin C, Yeh JL, Lin TM, Chai CY, Hsieh MW, Huang SH. Autologous fat grafting in female genital area improves sexual function by increasing Collagenesis, angiogenesis, and estrogen receptors. Aesthetic Surg J 2023.
4. Padoin AV, Braga-Silva J, Martins P, et al. Sources of processed lipoaspirate cells: influence of donor site on cell concentration. Plast Reconstr Surg. 2008;122:614–8.
5. Moore JH Jr, Kolaczynski JW, Morales LM, et al. Viability of fat obtained by syringe suction lipectomy: effects of local anesthesia with lidocaine. Aesth Plast Surg. 1995;194:335–9.
6. Eto H, Kato H, Suga H, et al. The fate of adipocytes after nonvascularized fat grafting: evidence of early death and replacement of adipocytes. Plast Reconstr Surg. 2012;1295:1081–92.

7. Kurita M, Matsumoto D, Shigeura T, et al. Influences of centrifugation on cells and tissues in liposuction aspirates: optimized centrifugation for lipotransfer and cell isolation. Plast Reconstr Surg. 2008;1213:1033–1041; discussion 1042-–1033.
8. Smith OJ, Jell G, Mosahebi A. The use of fat grafting and platelet-rich plasma for wound healing: a review of the current evidence. Int Wound J. 2019;16(1):275–85. https://doi.org/10.1111/iwj.13029. Epub 2018 Nov 20. PMID: 30460739; PMCID: PMC7948810.
9. Vogt PM, Herold C, Rennekampff HO. Autologous fat transplantation for labia majora reconstruction. Aesth Plast Surg. 2011;35(5):913–5. https://doi.org/10.1007/s00266-011-9664-5. Epub 2011 Feb 27.
10. Lin JY, Wang C, Pu LL. Can we standardize the techniques for fat grafting? Clin Plast Surg. 2015;42(2):199–208. https://doi.org/10.1016/j.cps.2014.12.005. Epub 2015 Feb 20.

Chapter 15
Role of Biomaterials for the Approach of Labia Majora Aesthetic and Functional Alterations

Pablo Gonzalez Isaza

A biomaterial is any compound, natural or synthetic, that can be used in the human body to augment or enhance tissues, and it can also have bio-stimulative properties according to its components. There are many options that come from aesthetic medicine practice and have migrated to be used in the genital area.

The main compounds can be divided into 1. collagen bio-stimulators, 2. fillers, and 3. threads.

Collagen bio-stimulators are substances that are injected near the dermal layer to generate a controlled inflammatory process in the tissues with the posterior migration of fibroblasts and macrophages that modify the ground matrix and consequently stimulate the production of collagen I–III.

These compounds have been traditionally used in face and body with excellent results and a very low rate of complications and now are used for labia majora enhancement under off-label indications; besides collagen stimulation, these compounds increase skin quality, luminosity, and humidity, and dilutions and concentrations vary according to the indications, but in general aesthetic goals are met without known serious side effects (Fig. 15.1a, b).

The most common collagen bio-stimulators are PLLA (polylactic acid), calcium hydroxyapatite, and PDO (polydioxanone).

P. Gonzalez Isaza (✉)
Obstetrics and Gynecology, Urogynecology Minimally Invasive Surgery, Hospital Universitario San Jorge, Pereira, Colombia

Soranus Center for Funtional and Regenerative Urogynecology, Pereira, Colombia

P. Gonzalez Isaza (ed.), *Aesthetic and Functional Alterations of the Labia Majora*, https://doi.org/10.1007/978-3-031-97405-2_15

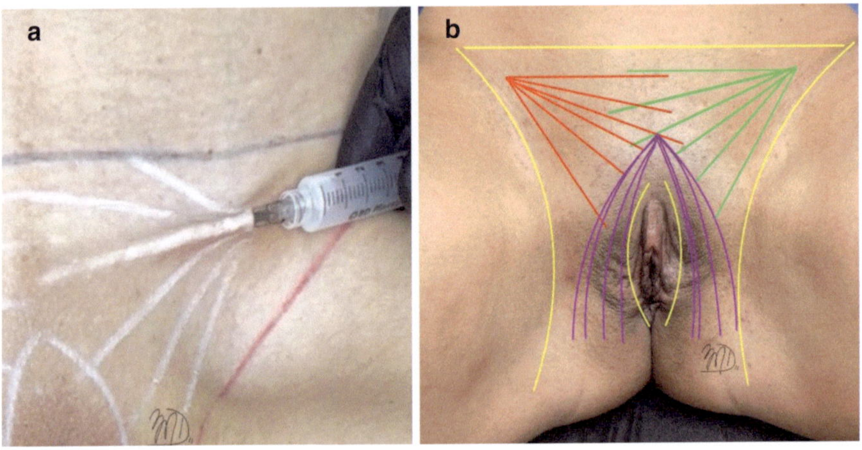

Fig. 15.1 (**a**, **b**) Example of Biomaterials PLLA (poly-L-lactic acid) Injection. (Courtesy: Dr. Mariana Montoya, personal experience)

15.1 Mechanism of Action

1. Poly-L-lactic acid is a synthetic material biodegradable, biocompatible derived from sugar fermentation, and converted into small particles of 40–63 microns. When injected inside superficial dermis, these particles induce a cytokine and growth factors-mediated inflammatory response, which attract fibroblasts and keratinocytes that are responsible for collagen production and improvement of skin quality inside a regenerative environment.

Tissue macrophages break down the poly-L-lactic acid into lactic acid monomers, which are metabolized to carbon dioxide and water while stimulating the production of new collagen type-I fibers in the skin, and half of the product is digested within 6 months. The effect can last up to 24 months [1–3]. The degradation of PLLA is a complex process through the production of enzymes by neutrophils, macrophages, and fibroblasts such as acid phosphatase and lactate dehydrogenase [4].

Inside our center we mostly use (PLLA) in a non-pyrogenic solution containing 150 mg 90 mg carboxymethylcellulose 127,5 mg mannitol we dilute it with 18 cc Normal saline and 2 cc of 2%lidocaine without epinephrine, 20 cc of solution are carefully injected around mons pubis and labia majora,0.1 CC X CM2 of skin for skin tightening and 0.2 CC X CM2 of skin for a volumizing effect (Fig. 15.1a, b). We consider this product a potent and effective collagen bio-stimulator, for cases where there is mild to moderate skin laxity, according to the pinch test (Fig. 15.2a, b).

Another collagen bio-stimulator is calcium hydroxyapatite (Ca Ha) is commonly found in bone and teeth with natural metabolism and excretion. When it is used inside fillers, different concentrations and suspension mediums can be found, and the most important effects are collagenesis skin tightening and volumization, without migration of the product.

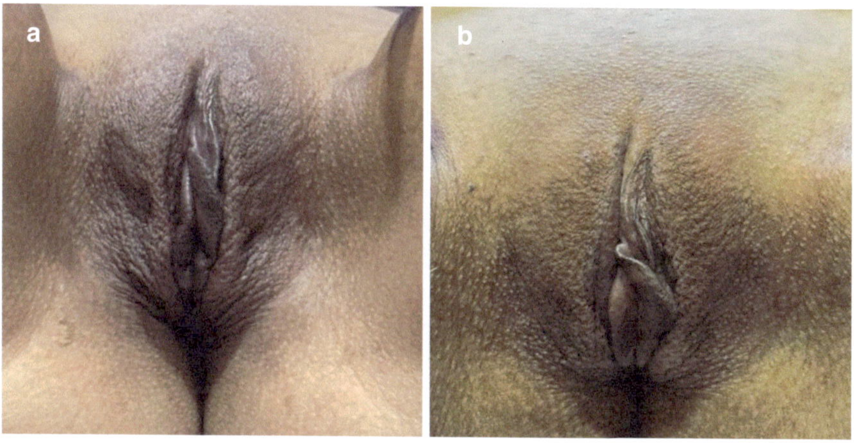

Fig. 15.2 (**a**) Before PLLA injection (poly-L-lactic acid). (**b**) 45 days after PLLA injection

A recent randomized controlled trial by Vilela et al. compared calcium hydroxy-apatite against hyaluronic acid injection and found similar results when used for labia majora atrophic conditions regarding safety and efficacy [5].

15.2 Fillers

The most common fillers are based on cross-linked hyaluronic acid; inside our center we have tested many brands, with different properties, regarding cross-linking agent, density, and rheological properties (Table 15.1). From 2015 to 2016, we participated inside research of 37 patients suffering from labia majora hypotrophy, hyaluronic acid hydrogel 28 mg/mL (PEG) polyethylene-glycol cross-linked (Neauvia Intense Rose Matex Lab Switzerland) was used.

The protocol involved the injection of 1.0–1.5 cc of the product at the level of each labia majora between the fascia of dartos and the fibrous tunic containing the adipose body (Figs. 15.3–15.7).

Patients reported high satisfaction with labia majora volume up to 12 months after the injection, the procedure was very safe, and the patient's complaints were related to temporary pain and minimal swelling 3–5 days after the injection [6].

Another product that we have used for many years as a labia majora volumizer is based on BDD (1,4-Butanediol diglycidyl ether) cross-linked 21 mg/mL hyaluronic Desirial Plus (Vivacy Inc., France) (Figs. 15.8–15.11). The protocol involved the injection of 1.0 cc of the product at the level of each labia majora between the fascia of Dartos and the fibrous tunic containing the adipose body.

Patients reported high satisfaction with labia majora volume up to 14 months after the injection, and we found quite interesting rheological properties regarding a delicate balance of viscosity/elasticity/density, which demonstrated very good aesthetic results lasting up to 10 months, with very low side effects and a high safety profile.

Table 15.1 Different methods for labia majora aesthetic and functional alterations approach

Component	Characteristics	Protocols	Clinical effects	Lasting effect	Complications
Polylactic acid (PLLA)	Collagen stimulator Microparticles (40–63 microns) Biocompatible Biodegradable	One application 2 months apart three sessions	Skin tightening brightness Volumizing effect	18 months	Foreign body reaction Granuloma Allergies Asymmetries Transitory pain
Calcium hydroxyapatite	Collagen stimulator Microspheres (20–45 microns) similar to bone components	One application 6–12 months apart	Can improve skin quality, tightening effect Volumizing effect	12–15 months	Inflammation erythema pain hematomas migration asymmetry vascular occlusion
Hyaluronic acid PEG glycated	Filler Volumization	One application 6–18 months apart	Skin hydration volumizing effect Can improve skin quality	6–18 months	Edema erythema granuloma Reversible with hyaluronidase
Hyaluronic acid BDDE cross-linked	Filler volumization Absorbable biocompatible	One application 6–10 months apart	Skin hydration volumizing effect Can improve skin quality	6–10 months	Foreign body reaction Granuloma Fibrotic reaction
Suspension threads PCL	Lifting method Antiaging effect Tissue revitalization	One application 18–24 months apart	Soft tissue suspension	18–24 months	Foreign body reaction Granuloma Extrusion Infection
Suspension threads PDO Collagen stimulation Synthetic polydioxanone polymer Biocompatible Biodegradable					
Stimulation threads PLLA	Antiaging effect Tissue revitalization	One application 6–10 months apart	Skin hydration volumizing effect Can improve skin quality	6–10 months	Foreign body reaction Granuloma Extrusion Infection

PEG polyethylene-glycol (cross-linking agent), *BDDE* 1,4-Butanediol diglycidyl ether (cross-linking agent), *PCL* polycaprolactone (thread material), *PDO*: polydioxanone (thread material), *PLLA*: polylactic acid (thread material)

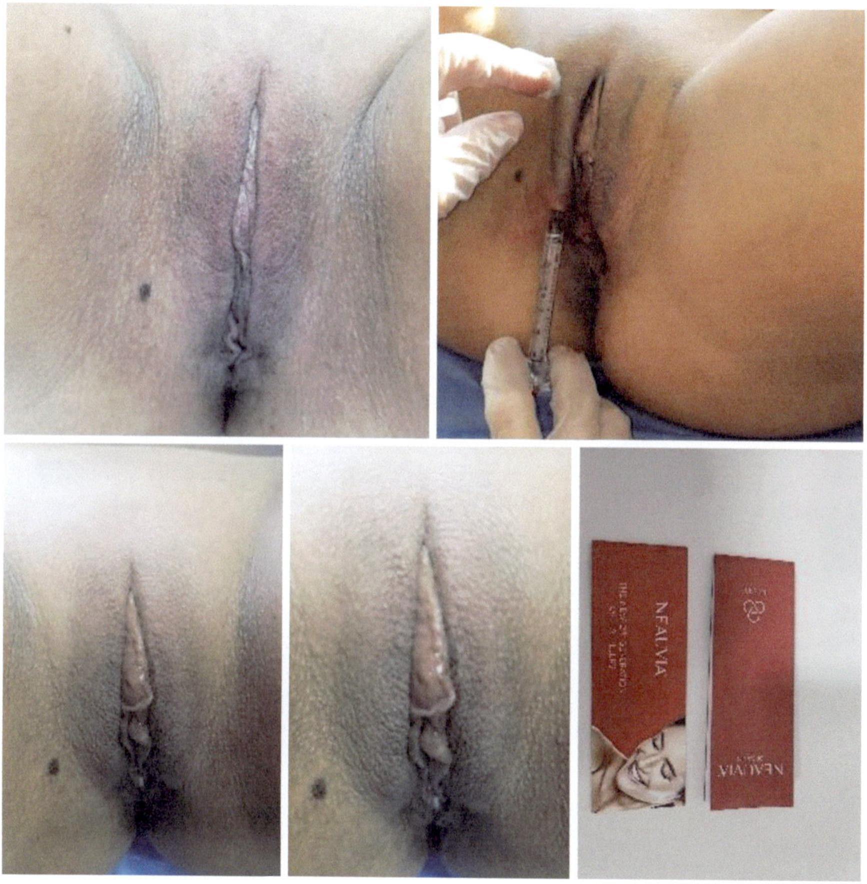

Figs. 15.3–15.7 Technique of application (before, immediate after, 1 month, 3 months and after injection)

Another indication for the use of this product with a lower concentration and special rheological features is for chronic vulvar and perineal fissures. The site of injection is at the level of vulvar vestibule and perineal body skin, topical anesthesia lidocaine 20% tetracaine 10% is applied by the patients 40 minutes before the injection. The area is cleaned with iodine solution, before the injection is performed, a standardized technique of injection is used by delivering 0.2–0.3 mL of the precharged product with a 30-gauge needle around vulvar vestibule and perineal body skin, and a gauge impregnated with antibiotic solution is left inside vagina for 6 hours and removed at home; patients are encouraged to stop sexual intercourse for 5–7 days after the injection, office setting easy and reproducible procedure. It is also a safe and effective nonhormonal alternative for the improvement of symptoms of

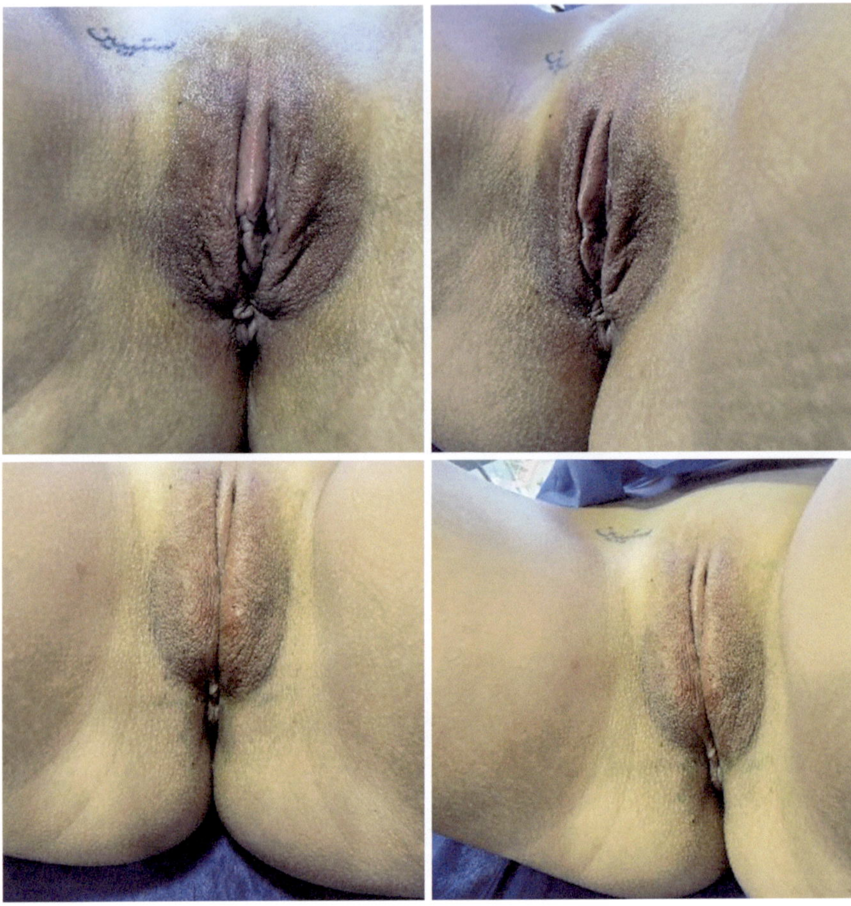

Figs 15.8–15.11 Before and after injection

affected women with this painful condition, and it can last up to 9 months and can be repeated once the effect is over. Cross-linked hyaluronic acid injections offer a longer effect, improving trophism, vestibule elasticity, and dispersion of superficial nerve endings, breaking the cycle of formation of fissures at the level of posterior fourchette (Figs. 15.12–15.14) [7].

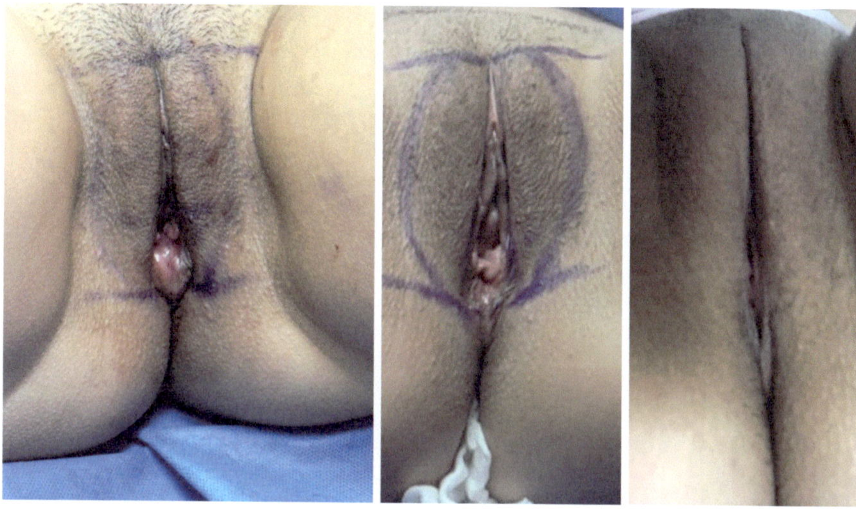

Figs. 15.12–15.14 Before and after injection

15.3 Threads

Thread lifting has widely been used in aesthetic medicine. Its main principle is related to mechanotransduction, which is the ability of the cell to sense, process, and respond to mechanical stimuli, and is an important regulator of physiologic function, which has been found to play a role in regulating gene expression, protein synthesis, cell differentiation, and tissue growth [8].

Threads are always a good option either for suspension or for collagen stimulation; there are different types of threads regarding composition material and physical characteristics of the thread itself, barbed, not barbed, net configuration, etc (Table 15.2).

Most of the methods for thread lifting involve the movement of soft tissues in a direction opposite or perpendicular to the vectors of tissue ptosis.

The basic principle of thread lifting is to bring one tissue closer to another; it is also possible to add volume.

All threads for lifting or bio-stimulation are composed of materials existing in suturing for surgery.

Absorbable threads contain polylactic acid, polycaprolactone, and hyaluronic acid in their structure, which stimulate the synthesis of collagen and elastin, as well as neo angiogenesis (Figs. 15.15 and 15.16).

Table 15.2 Different materials used in threads for labia majora aesthetic and functional alterations

	Polydioxanone (PDO)	Polylactic acid (PLLA)	Polycaprolactone (PCL)
Biodegradation period	6–8 months	14–18 months	16–24 months
Flexibility	Average	Low	High
Discomfort	Slight	Strong	No discomfort
Hydrolitic resolution	Average	Average	High
Safety	High	High	High

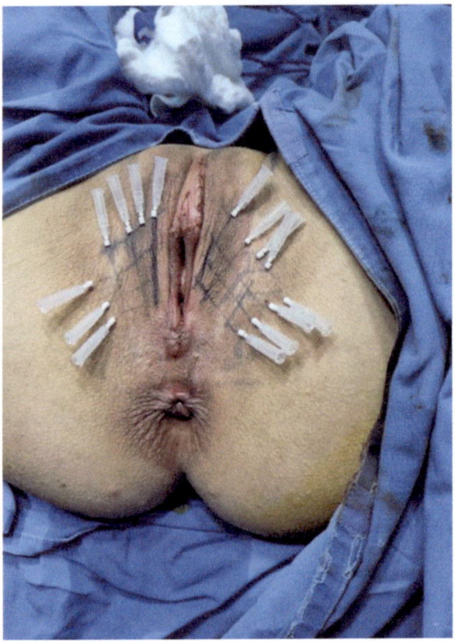

Fig. 15.15 Collagen stimulation threads

Inside our unit we have tested different brands of threads, and its use has been more focused for face or body treatments, but for genitals, there is scarce information inside the scientific literature, regarding safety and effectiveness for genital use.

According to our algorithmic approach for labia majora aesthetic and functional complaints, we decide to use threads for selected cases of labia majora skin laxity conditions, either as a monotherapy or in combination with fillers or energy-based devices like bipolar, fractional, or dielectric radiofrequency (Table 15.3).

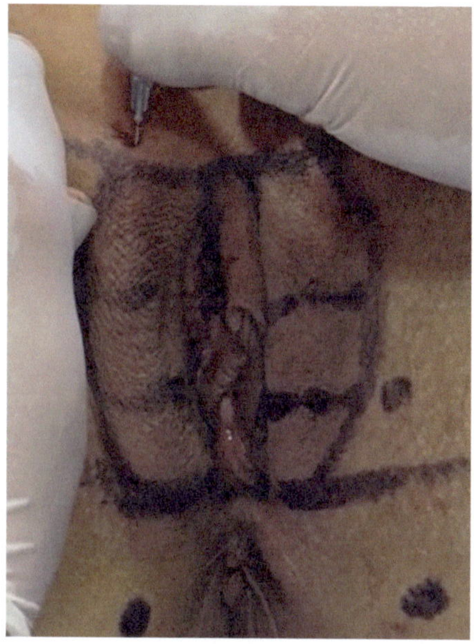

Fig. 15.16 Suspension threads

Table 15.3 Algorithmic approach for labia majora aesthetic and functional alterations

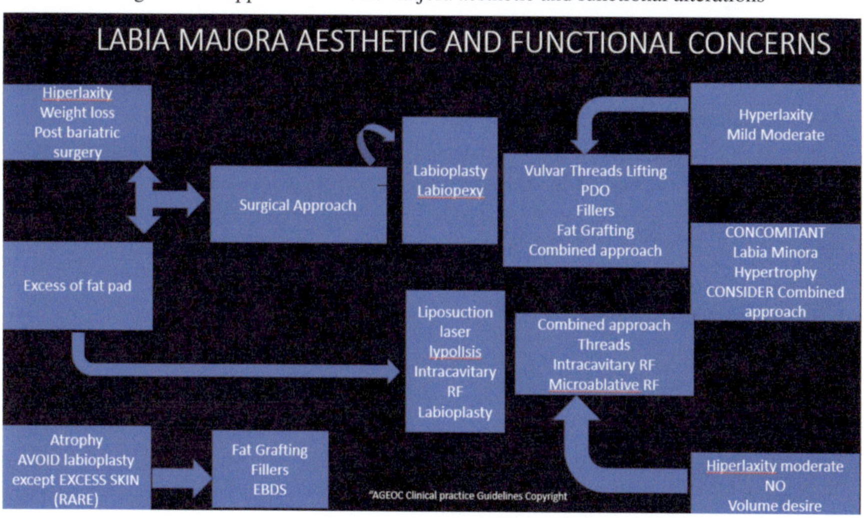

15.4 Important Comments

It is always important to remark that any product to be injected into labia majora as a volumizer or vaginal mucosa for hydration must comply with local health regulations, which can assure that these types of products are safe and effective in the genital area.

Unfortunately, most of the complications reported regarding injections of hyaluronic acid are related to the use of products designed for face and body, with different rheological properties, not optimal for these delicate areas.

15.5 Complications

Any biomaterial injected or inserted inside soft human body tissues can have side effects such as edema, erythema rejection, infection, migration, and even allergic reactions.

There are important aspects to consider when using these materials, such as their origin quality, histological studies, and also safety and effectiveness studies.

A complete clinical file can rule out previous reactions with biomaterials, so a wise decision should be made to exclude these patients.

Nowadays most companies that produce biomaterials work hard to offer high quality biocompatible products that can be used safely with low rate of side effects.

Biomaterials are traditionally used for face and body treatments, and it is important to remark that any compound or material should comply with health regulations to be used in the genital area; otherwise the use is considered off-label, and a good example of this is related to the rheological properties of hyaluronic acid-based fillers as volumizing alternatives for labia majora that should support mechanical forces such as intercourse and specific exercises (horseback riding and bicycle riding among others) that could lead to a faster absorption of the biomaterial.

References

1. Herrmann JL, Hoffmann RK, Ward CE, Schulman JM, Grekin RC. Biochemistry, physiology, and tissue interactions of contemporary biodegradable injectable dermal fillers. Dermatologic Surg. 2018;44(Suppl 1):S19–31. [PubMed]
2. Hotta TA. Attention to infection prevention in medical aesthetic clinics. Plast Surg Nurs. 2018;38(1):17–24. [PubMed]
3. Pascali M, Quarato D, Carinci F. Filling procedures for lip and perioral rejuvenation: a systematic review. Rejuvenation Res. 2018;21(6):553–9. [PubMed]
4. da Silva D, Kaduri M, Poley M, Adir O, Krinsky N, Shainsky-Roitman J, Schroeder A. Biocompatibility, biodegradation and excretion of polylactic acid (PLA) in medical implants and theranostic systems. Chem. Eng J. 2018;15(340):9–14. [PMC free article] [PubMed]

5. Vilela CL, de Lima Faria GE, Boggio RF. Treatment of atrophy of the labia Majora: calcium hydroxyapatite or hyaluronic acid? Aesth Plast Surg. 2024;48(3):472–7. https://doi.org/10.1007/s00266-023-03617-3. Epub 2023 Sep 6. PMID: 37673803.
6. Zerbinati N, Lotti T, Monticelli D, Rauso R, González-Isaza P, D'Este E, Calligaro A, Sommatis S, Maccario C, Mocchi R, Lotti J, Wollina U, Tchernev G, França K. *In vitro* evaluation of the biosafety of hyaluronic acid PEG cross-linked with micromolecules of calcium hydroxyapatite in low concentration. Open Access Maced J Med Sci. 2018;6(1):15–9. https://doi.org/10.3889/oamjms.2018.044. PMID: 29483971; PMCID: PMC5816290
7. González-Isaza P, Sánchez-Prieto M, Sánchez-Borrego R. Chronic vulvar fissure: approach with cross-linked hyaluronic acid. Int Urogynecol J. 2023;34(7):1495–9. https://doi.org/10.1007/s00192-022-05401-4. Epub 2022 Nov 7. PMID: 36344691.
8. Shutova MS, Boehncke WH. Mechanotransduction in Skin Inflammation Cells. 2022;11(13):2026. https://doi.org/10.3390/cells11132026. PMID: 35805110; PMCID: PMC9265324.

Annexes

Labia Majora Treatments Gallery

Pablo González Isaza

(See Figs. A.1, A.2, A.3, A.4, A.5, A.6a, A.6b, A.7, A.8, A.9, and A.10)

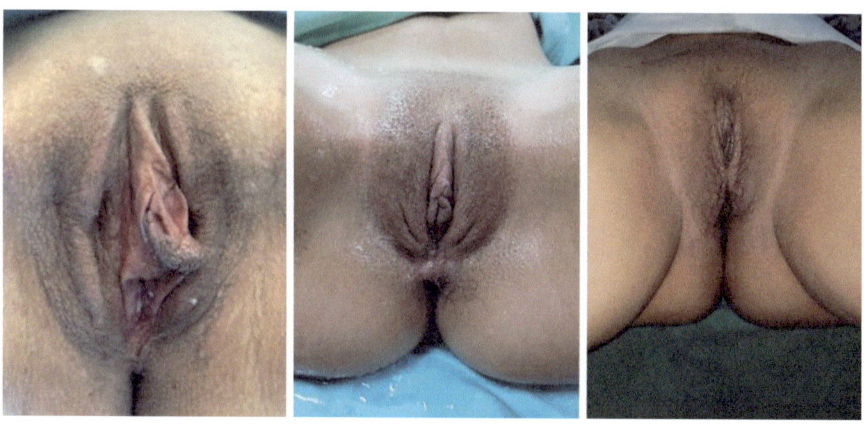

Fig. A.1 Cutaneous Hypelaxity (CHL) perineal generalized

P. Gonzalez Isaza (ed.), *Aesthetic and Functional Alterations of the Labia Majora*, https://doi.org/10.1007/978-3-031-97405-2

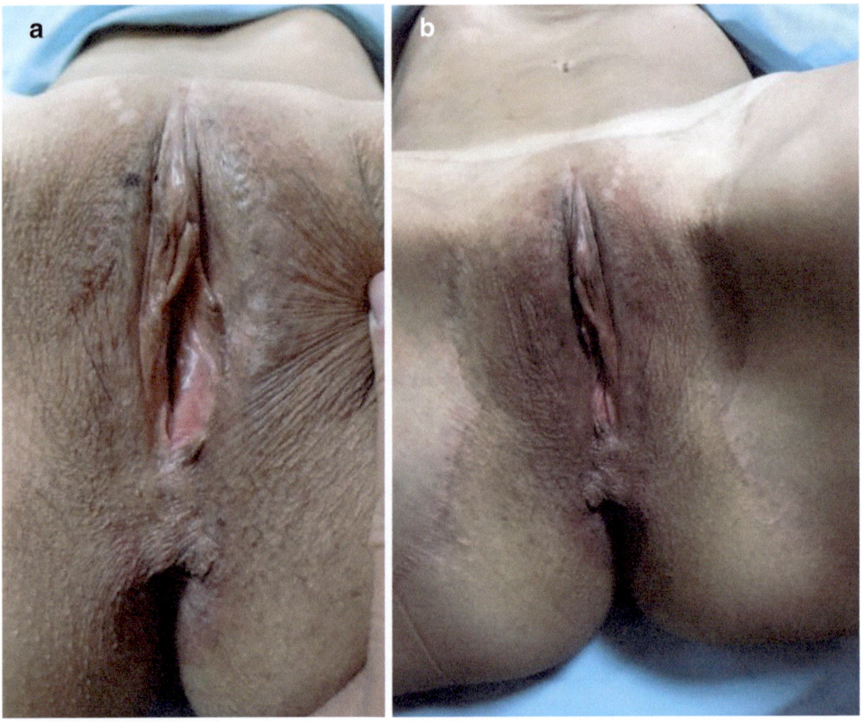

Fig. A.2 (**a, b**) Cutaneous Adipose Atrophy (CAA)

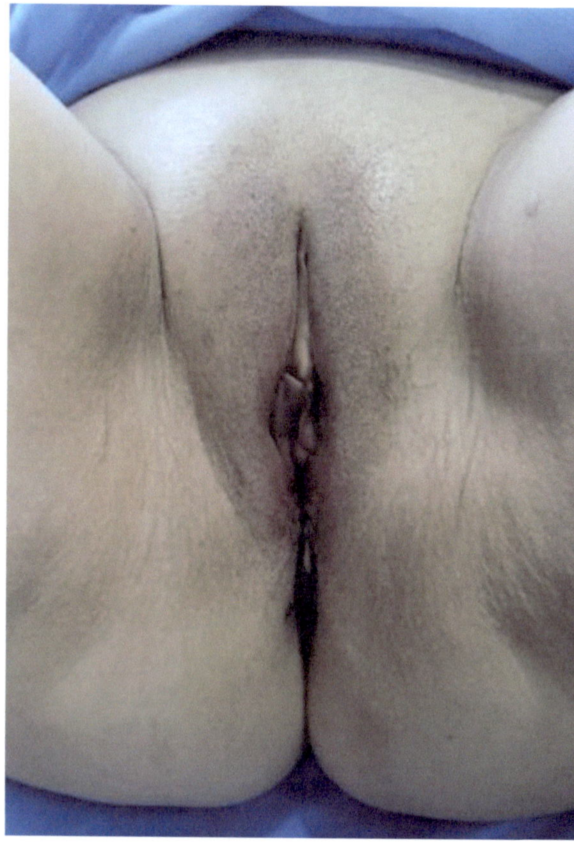

Fig. A.3 Adipose unilateral hypertrophy (congenital) (Chronic antiretroviral drug exposure)

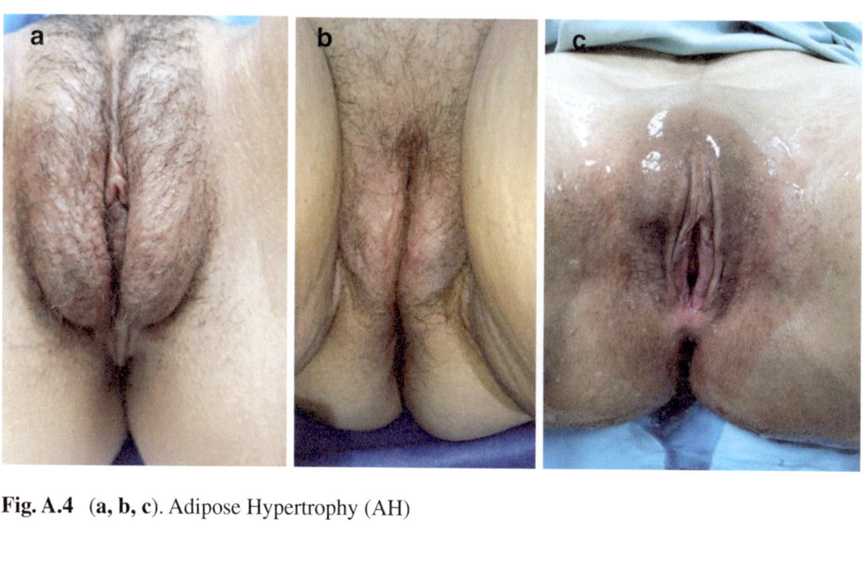

Fig. A.4 (**a, b, c**). Adipose Hypertrophy (AH)

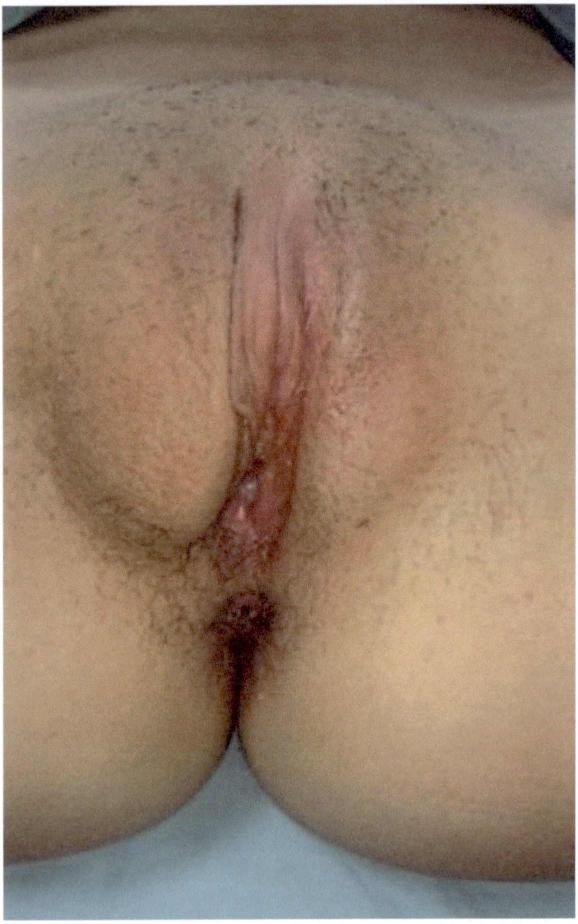

Fig. A.5 Adipose hypertrophy (congenital)

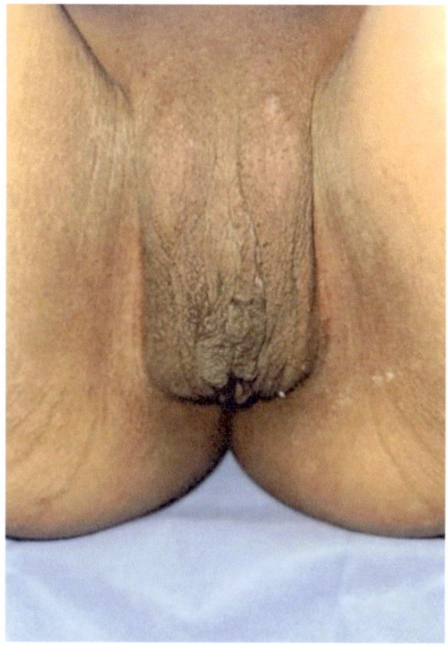

Fig. A.6a Iatrogenic conditions: (IC) (Iatrogenic filler volume)

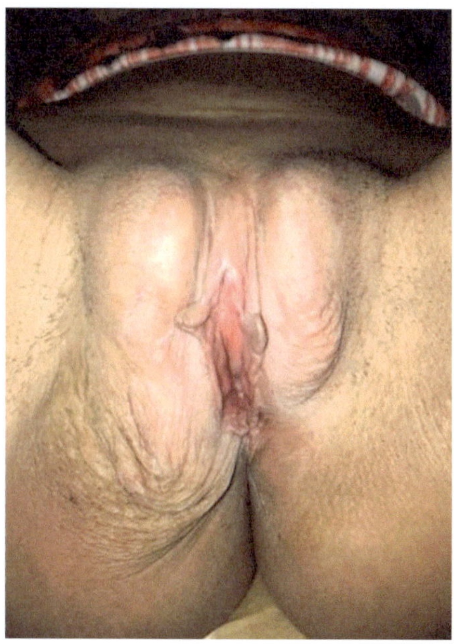

Fig. A.6b Iatrogenic conditions (IC) injection of silicone derivatives

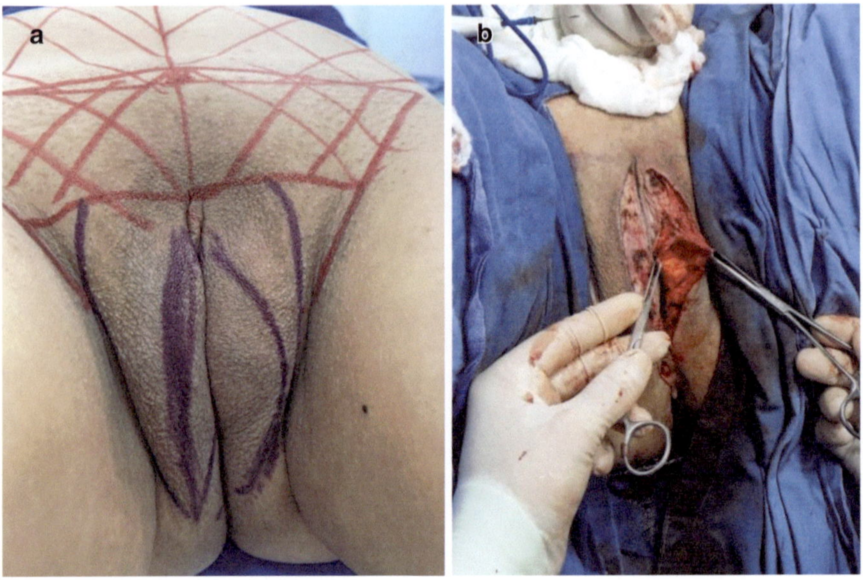

Fig. A.7 (**a**) Central unilateral lipodystrophy. (**b**) Dartos fascia site-specific defect

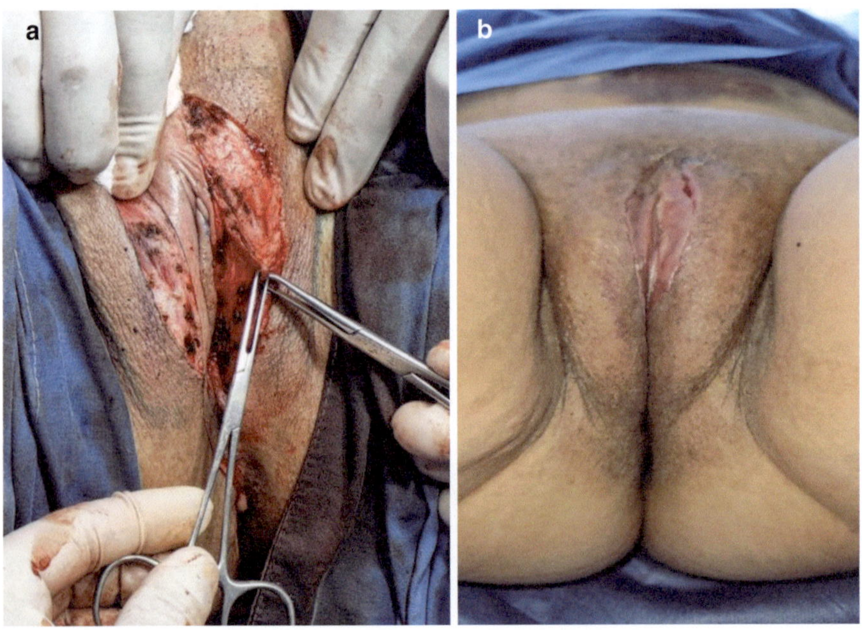

Fig. A.8 (**a**) Closure of dartos site-specific defect. (**b**) 8 days post-op

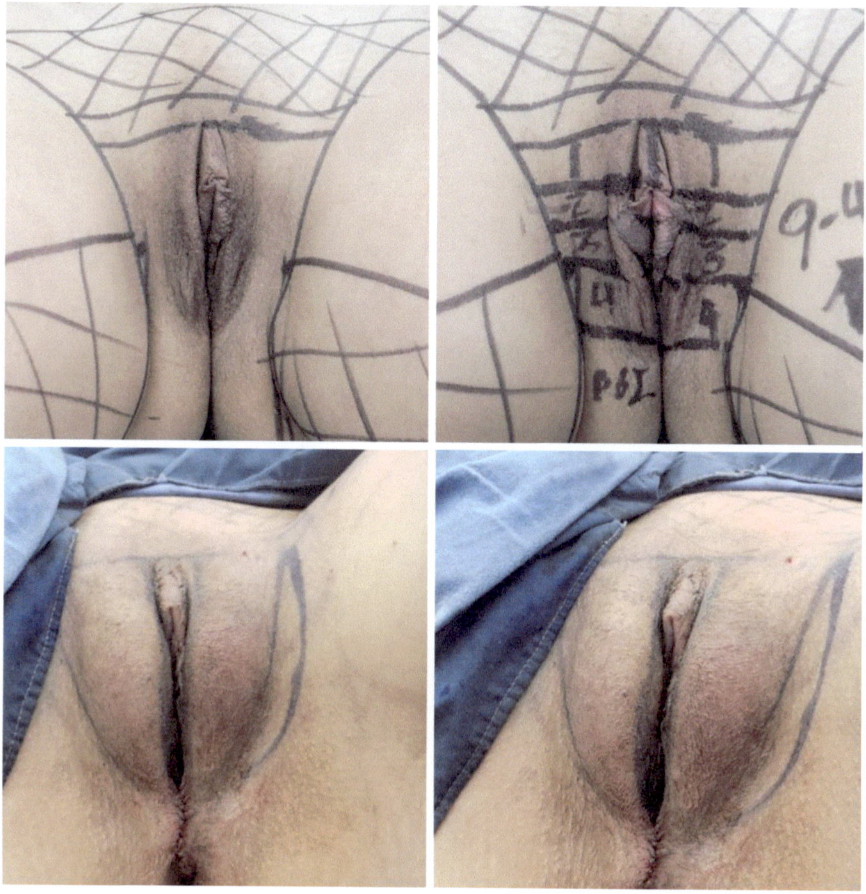

Fig. A.9 Combined labia minora labiaplasty/autologous fat grafting

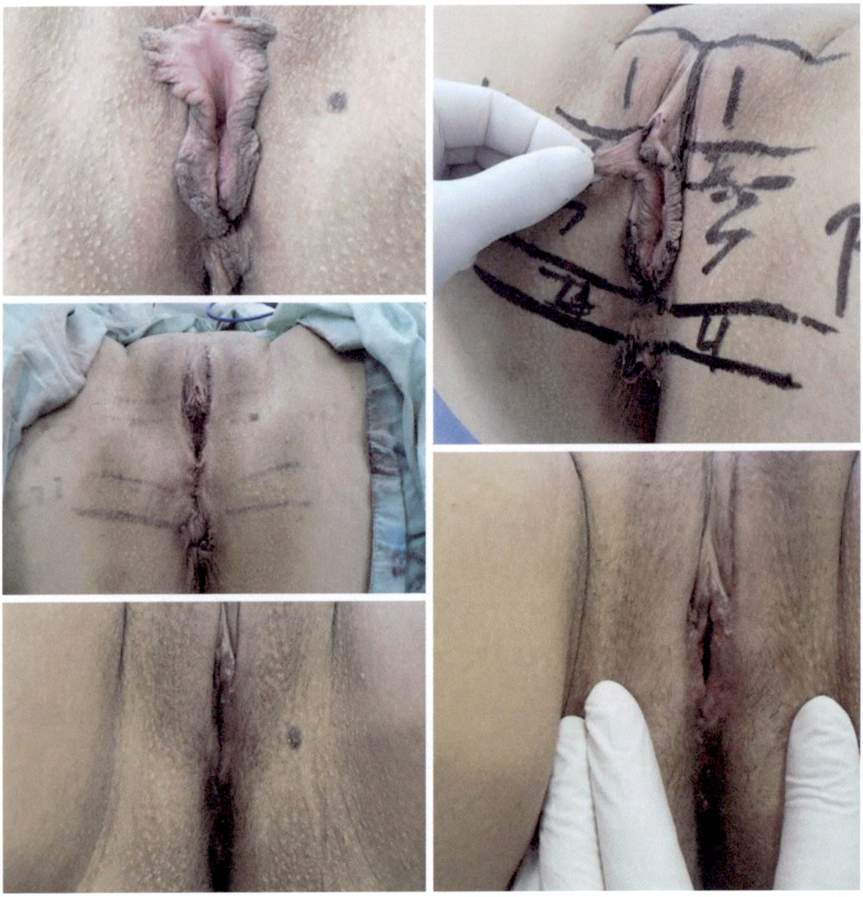

Fig. A.10 Botched labiaplasty reconstruction/cross-linked hyaluronic acid injection

Informed Consent

INFORMED CONSENT FOR MEDICAL PROCEDURES

AESTHETIC GYNECOLOGY

I ____ identified with ID number __________________

I will be performed by Dr. ------------------------ identification------------------------- medical record---------------------------------

____ Labiaplasty / Labia reduction (labia minora and/or labia majora).

____ Reduction of the clitoral hood /Reduction of the size of the clitoral hood.

____ Addressing Anatomical variants (accessory folds in labia clitoral hood) and perineal region.

____ Injection of filler materials in labia majora or vagina (Hyaluronic Acid cross-linked/non-cross-linked Platelet-rich plasma and/or growth factors) with aesthetic and/or functional purposes.

PLEASE READ THE FOLLOWING INFORMATION IN DETAIL.

I UNDERSTAND:

_____ 1. The risks of surgeries can be the following: prolonged or incomplete healing, surgical wound opening, irregularities, abnormal scarring or asymmetries in the size of the labia after surgery, infection, painful sexual intercourse, prolonged bleeding among other rare events.

_____ 2. The surgical area will be swollen, asymmetric and with possible color changes. In the weeks following the surgery, it may take 3 to 4 weeks to have an adequate recovery and 3 to 4 months to obtain the definitive aesthetic and/or functional results.

_____ 3. Sometimes it is necessary to perform a "**second surgical time or revision"** to reduce the size of the lips according to the aesthetic conformity and functionality. Most of the time this revision does not generate any type of charge with respect to medical fees, but it could generate minimal operating costs of materials, anesthesia, among others.

_____ 4. I agree to limit my physical and sexual activity for as long as indicated by the surgical conditions.

_____ 5. I understand that Dr. Pablo Gonzalez Isaza will use all his expertise and knowledge to balance aesthetics, functionality and conditions, but at no time can he guarantee perfect and surreal results.

_____ 6. Smoking patients have a higher risk of poor postoperative results and alterations in healing, and additionally a greater potential for infectious events and bleeding. **If you are a smoker, it is advisable to stop smoking 2 to 4 weeks before the surgical procedure,** but this is not a guarantee to avoid the potential complications previously exposed.

_____ 7. I certify that I have informed Dr. Pablo Gonzalez Isaza in a timely manner about my medical history and medical background. I understand that withholding information could lead to complications and risks during the surgical procedure.

_____ 8. In my own words, the following is what I want to get out of my surgical procedure by Dr:

____

____

____

____

_____ 9. I certify, that I have had a consultation with Dr. --, and all aspects of my surgical procedure have been properly explained to me.

_____ 10. I understand the procedure, its risks, complications and the recovery process. I agree to carefully follow all the instructions given by Dr. -- and his team, as well as I will report any eventuality that may occur during the recovery process.

_____ 11. I understand that I have received sufficient information in order to make the decision to undergo the surgical procedure. All questions have been answered.

_____ 12. Additionally, I authorize Dr. -------------------------------------- to make photographic and video recordings for medical record keeping purposes and may obtain a copy of this material upon request.

_____ 13. I authorize Dr. --------------------------------------a to use photographic and video material related to my surgical procedure, for purely academic and scientific research purposes, preserving at all times my identity and privacy.

_______________________ _______________

PATIENT SIGNATURE DATE

_______________________ _______________

TUTOR OR ASSISTANT DATE

___________________________ _______________

DR. ------------------------------------- DATE

Validated Questionnaires to Assess Aesthetic and Functional Aspects Before and After Labia Majora Treatments

COPS-L

COPS -L for Women Seeking Labiaplasty

GAS

Veale, David & Eshkevari, Ertimiss & Ellison, Nell & Cardozo, Linda & Robinson, Dudley & Kavouni, Angelica. (2013). Genetial Appearance Satisfaction Scale (Bramwell, 2009).

Below you will find a number of statements that women often make when referring to the genital area, read each one, and choose the answer that you feel applies to you. A diagram of the anatomy of the female external genitalia will be provided.

1. I feel that my genitals are normal looking.

   Never Sometimes Almost always Always

2. I feel that my genitals look unattractive.

   Never Sometimes Almost always Always

3. I feel my labia vulvae are too long.

   Never Sometimes Almost always Always

4. I am satisfied with the appearance of my genitals.

   Never Sometimes Almost always Always

5. I experience irritation of my labia when exercising or walking.

   Never Sometimes Almost always Always

6. I feel or have felt conscious of labia size in sexual situations because of the appearance of my genitals.

   Never Sometimes Almost always Always

7. I am embarrassed by the appearance of my genitals and it limits my enjoyment of sex.

Never Sometimes Almost always Always

8. I feel discomfort in my genitals when I wear tight clothing.

Never Sometimes Almost always Always

9. I feel that my genital area is visible through tight clothing.

Never Sometimes Almost always Always

10. I am concerned about the appearance of my genital area.

Never Sometimes Almost always Always

11. I feel that my genital area looks asymmetrical or larger on one side.

Never Sometimes Almost always Always

Index

P. Gonzalez Isaza (ed.), *Aesthetic and Functional Alterations of the Labia Majora*, https://doi.org/10.1007/978-3-031-97405-2

MIX
Papier aus verantwortungsvollen Quellen
Paper from responsible sources
FSC® C105338

If you have any concerns about our products,
you can contact us on
ProductSafety@springernature.com

In case Publisher is established outside the EU,
the EU authorized representative is:
Springer Nature Customer Service Center GmbH
Europaplatz 3, 69115 Heidelberg, Germany

Printed by Libri Plureos GmbH
in Hamburg, Germany